The Pocket Encyclopedia of

Prescription

and

Nonprescription

Drugs

Samuel Perry, M.D.

Simon and Schuster/New York

KEY TO SYMBOLS

|A| take with an antacid to reduce stomach irritation
|B| take at bedtime
|C| if taken with a caffeine source (coffee or tea) drowsiness may be reduced
|D| may cause psychological and physical dependence
|E| take at least 1 hour before eating
|F| take with or immediately following food to reduce stomach irritation
|I| intensifies the effect of alcohol
|P| take with a potassium-rich diet

Publishers Note

Drugs are simultaneously among the most remarkable and beneficial outgrowths of medical science as well as among the most abused and misused. The purpose of this guide is to acquaint the reader with the almost endless number of drugs available and to provide a ready source from which the reader can determine which drugs are generally used for what purposes, what alternative drugs are available for these purposes, and what side-effects a user of a particular drug might reasonably anticipate experiencing.

Of course, no general work can be expected to anticipate fully either the effectiveness or the potential side-effects any particular individual may experience in connection with their use of a drug. Accordingly, the Publishers can accept no responsibility for any consequences resulting from the use or reliance by the reader upon information contained herein.

Produced by Mitchell Beazley Publishers
87–89 Shaftesbury Avenue, London W1V 7 AD
Copyright © Mitchell Beazley Publishers 1981
Published by Simon and Schuster
A Division of Gulf & Western Corporation
Simon & Schuster Building
Rockefeller Center
1230 Avenue of the Americas
New York, New York 10020
SIMON AND SCHUSTER is a trademark of Simon & Schuster
Library of Congress Cataloging in Publication Data
Perry, Samuel.

    The Pocket Encyclopedia of Prescription and
    Nonprescription Drugs
    1. Drugs—Handbooks, manuals, etc.
    2. Pharmacology—Handbooks, manuals, etc.
    I. Title. [DNLM: 1. Drugs—Ency popu. 2. Drugs,
    Nonprescription—Encyclopedias, Popular.
    QV 13 P465p]
    RM300.P468   615'.1'0321   80-9061
    ISBN 0-671-42398-3   AACR1

Editor: Susan Carter Elliott
Assistant Editors: Suzanne S. Burke, Carolyn Westberg
Executive Editor: Hal Robinson
Editor-in-Chief: Susannah Read
Typeset by Mim-G Studios, Inc.
Printed in the United States of America

CONTENTS

INTRODUCTION

The more you know about the medicine you are taking, the better your chances of using the medicine effectively and safely. To make this information conveniently accessible, *The Pocket Encyclopedia of Prescription and Nonprescription Drugs* is designed to fit in your medicine cabinet and to be carried in your pocket or purse when you go to consult your doctor or to obtain drugs from the pharmacy.

Over 400 of the most frequently prescribed medicines are discussed along with more than 300 common nonprescription drugs sold "over the counter" (OTC). To learn about the medicine you are taking, first look it up in the index and then turn to the page where your drug is described. You will see that the description for each drug has several parts:

- Name of the drug (generic and brand names)

- Dosage form (capsule, tablet, liquid, lotion, etc.)

- Indications (what problem the drug treats)

- Actions (what the drug does)

- Possible side effects (mild and severe)

- Special instructions on how and when to take the drug (for example, with milk, before meals, etc.)

- Special warnings

- *Name of the Drug.* Every medicine is listed under the official *generic* name (for example, penicillin), then the manufacturers'*brand* names (Pen-Vee K, or V-Cillin K). Because your doctor or pharmacist may have used either the generic or brand name, *both* are listed in the index. For example, if you look up the brand name Librium in the index, you will be properly referred to the generic name chlordiazepoxide. (Of note, the generic name of your drug is worth knowing because some drugs can be ordered by generic instead of brand names and are often less expensive and just as effective.)

Some medicines contain more than one active ingredient. These *combination drugs* also appear in the index under both the generic and brand names. For example, a common abdominal relaxant is listed under both the generic name phenobarbital, hyoscyamine sulfate, atropine sulfate, hyoscine hydrobromide and under the brand name Donnatal. Along with reading about the combination drug, you may wish to look up separately the different active ingredients (such as phenobarbital) to acquire even more information about the combination drug's potential actions or side effects.

- *Dosage Form.* Medicines sometimes are available in more than one form. Of course, not all dosage forms have the same effect, so your doctor will decide which form to prescribe. Young children, for example, are frequently given a liquid antibiotic because it is easier to swallow, while an adult will usually prefer the convenience of the capsule or pill.

- *Indications:* The approved reasons for taking the drug

are listed (for example, heartbeat irregularities, eye infection, diabetes, etc.).

- *Actions:* A simplified statement explains how the drug produces its therapeutic effect (for example, regulates heartbeat, kills bacteria, lowers blood sugar, etc.).

- *Possible Side Effects.* All drugs can produce both wanted and unwanted effects. Some unwanted effects are simply annoying but expected reactions that occur "on the side." The severity of these *side effects* varies depending on the individual, the dosage, and the circumstances, but generally they are tolerable and can be regarded as the price one must pay for the therapeutic effect. For example, the drowsiness produced by many decongestants is inconvenient but not often a reason to discontinue the medicine. In this book, a drug's predictable side effects are listed so you are aware but not alarmed when these unwanted but relatively harmless reactions occur.

- A more serious type of unwanted drug effect is called an *adverse reaction.* If you experience such an infrequent but potentially harmful reaction, you should contact your doctor as soon as possible and perhaps discontinue the medication. The line between side effect and adverse reaction is not always easily drawn, however, and in every case where you have any doubt about the effect of a drug, it is very important that you consult your doctor. In this book, possible adverse reactions to the listed drug are in italics so you will know which reactions can be more serious. Furthermore, an asterisk placed next to a medical term indicates that it is one of many that have been defined in the glossary section, Medical and Drug Terms.

- *How and When to Take the Drug.* Some medicines are more effective if taken in a special way. For example, penicillin G should not be taken with food whereas the hormone prednisone should always be taken with meals. In this book the listed drug will have a symbol to indicate if there are any special instructions about its administration (see Key to Symbols at the front of the book).

- *Warning.* This final item of the drug listing will point out potential known hazards of the drug, such as an association with birth defects or a suspected carcinogen. Any drug is potentially hazardous. In a susceptible individual, one tablet of penicillin may cause a fatal allergic reaction—even a couple of aspirin may cause a bleeding ulcer. Although these severe reactions are not always predictable, many dangers can be avoided if both the doctor and the drug consumer (i.e. you) are well informed. This book provides information that may be of help in preventing a serious problem related to drug usage.

- *Drug Record.* A Patient's Prescription and Immunization Record is provided on Page 136. On this chart you can list any drugs you are currently taking, adverse or allergic reactions, and recent immunizations. There is a space to record the date, purpose, and prescribing doctor, as well as the pharmacy prescription number. You may also wish to make a personal notation beside the drug entry about your experience taking the drug, including comments about the drug's therapeutic and side effects. This information should be given to your prescribing doctor. He or she will need to know what drugs you are taking currently, as there are some drugs that should not be taken together because they interact unfavorably.

• It is particularly important to note any allergic reaction you might have had to a particular drug. Even if you are not specifically asked, you should tell the doctor about these reactions. The doctor should also know if you are allergic by nature. Sometimes, particularly when ill, people cannot recall exactly what allergic reaction was associated with which drug. For this reason you may wish to bring the pocket encyclopedia with you to the doctor's office. Remember, even a minor rash when taking a drug may be an indication that a more severe allergic reaction will occur if the drug is continued or taken again. Also, two seemingly unrelated drugs may be "cross sensitive," which means that an allergic reaction to one indicates a likely allergic reaction to the other.

• *Nonprescription Medicine.* Some people mistakenly believe that drugs not requiring a doctor's prescription are safe and are not "real" drugs. In fact, drugs sold "over the counter" (OTC) can cause serious problems; for example, an overdosage of many popular decongestants can cause psychosis, fever, seizures, coma, and death. With nonprescription medicine the drug consumer (you) and not the doctor must often determine how the drug should be taken and if the potential therapeutic benefits from the drug outweigh the potential risks.

Because all manufacturers of nonprescription drugs are required by law to enclose information about the drug's dosage, indications, and dangers, a detailed description has not been provided in this book. You should read the drug information on or inside the package carefully, paying special attention to parts labeled "warning" or "cautions," which may mean that for you the drug is "contraindicated." (Contraindications are conditions or situations that prohibit the use of a drug.) Recently, drug manufacturers have been required to distribute information about certain prescription medicines as well, such as tranquilizers. Your pharmacist will tell you which drugs have this requirement and, upon request, will give you the drug information pamphlet.

• *Disease Categories.* A particularly important feature of this book is that the prescription and nonprescription drugs are listed under different disease categories, such as Eyes, Infection, Pain, Nervous System, or Skin, Hair, and Scalp. For example, if you are having heart trouble, you can look in the index and learn that your medications are in the section entitled "Cardiovascular System." That section will introduce you to the kinds of drugs used for the heart as well as to special precautions you should take. The section will then list the common drugs you and your doctor may be using or may have considered using for your heart problem. Drugs used for more than one disease category are listed in the section of most common usage and cross-referenced in other sections. The index also lists symptoms, so that, for instance, you can locate the chapter that deals with respiratory medication by looking up "cough."

MEDICAL AND DRUG TERMS

abrasion—a wound resulting from scraping of the skin.

acute—of sudden onset, short-lived, not chronic.

addiction—the compulsive use of drugs or alcohol, without which the user would suffer physical or psychological trauma.

adverse reaction—harmful effect of a drug, not typical or expected.

allergen—any substance that induces an allergic reaction.

allergic reaction—the body's response to an allergen; may be mild or very severe (anaphylactic reaction); symptoms can include itching, skin rash, hives, sneezing, cough, asthma, feeling of suffocation, headache, throbbing in ears, convulsions, and sometimes death.

allergy—an abnormal sensitivity to a substance, such as a drug, that can develop gradually or suddenly.

amphetamine—a central nervous system stimulant.

analgesic—a pain-relieving remedy or drug.

anemia—a condition in which there is a diminished number of red blood cells to carry oxygen to body tissues.

anesthetic—a drug used to eliminate physical sensation either by loss of consciousness (general anesthesia) or by local application (topical anesthesia).

angina (or **angina pectoris**)—a feeling of suffocation and pressing chest pain caused by a decreased blood supply to the heart muscles; often triggered by excitement or exertion.

anorexia—extreme or prolonged loss of appetite.

antacid—an agent that neutralizes or reduces acidity in the stomach.

anti- —a prefix meaning counteractive or preventive, such as in antidepressant.

antibacterial—inhibiting the growth or spread of bacteria.

antibiotic—a substance that kills bacteria and other microorganisms or that prevents their spread or reproduction.

anticoagulant—an agent that retards the clotting or coagulation of blood.

anticonvulsant—a drug that controls seizures.

antidepressant—a drug that relieves depression.

antidote—a substance used to counter the effects of poison or other harmful conditions.

antifungal—an agent that counteracts fungi that cause infections.

antihistamine—a drug used to control allergic disorders or colds by counteracting the release of histamine in the body.

antipyretic—a drug that reduces fever, such as aspirin or acetaminophen.

antiseptic—an agent that reduces microorganisms on living tissue or other surfaces.

antispasmodic—a drug that reduces muscle spasms.

antitussive—a drug that reduces coughing.

arteriosclerosis—a condition that restricts blood flow as the vessel walls become thick and less elastic ("hardening of the arteries").

astringent—a substance that reduces secretions or bleeding by constricting blood vessels.

barbiturate—a compound derived from barbituric acid used for sedation or to induce sleep.

black tongue—a dark spot with thickened skin on the front of the tongue.

bladder disorder—abnormal condition of the receptacle that retains urine before elimination from the body; symptoms can include pain or burning upon urination, frequency, hesitancy, urgency, lack of urine, or inability to control urination (incontinence).

blood disorders—a decrease or malfunction of red blood cells, white blood cells, or platelets; can occur as an adverse reaction to certain drugs, chemicals, or radiation; symptoms can include anemia with resulting weakness, susceptibility to infections such as sore throats and pneumonia, and poor clotting with easy bruising or nosebleeds.

bone marrow depression—failure of the bone marrow to produce blood cells.

brand name—the registered term used by manufacturers to designate goods sold by them.

bronchial asthma—a respiratory disorder, often allergic and inherited, in which breathing becomes difficult due to spasms of the small breathing tubes.

buffered—relating to agents that protect against acidity.

carcinogen—any substance or condition known to increase the risk of cancer in humans and animals.

central nervous system—the brain and spinal cord.

chemotherapy—the treatment of disease with drugs.

compound—any combination of two or more ingredients.

congestion—fluid build-up caused by swollen tissue linings that restrict drainage and breathing.

contraceptive—a drug, device, or method used for birth control.

contraindication—a reason for a certain drug not to be used.

corticosteroids—hormone-like drugs that are used to treat allergies or inflammations.

cortisone—a commonly used corticosteroid.

decongestant—an agent that reduces congestion.

depressant—any drug, including alcohol, that reduces the activity of the central nervous system.

detoxify—to remove poisons or drugs from the body, or to reduce their harmful effects.

diabetes mellitus—a metabolic disorder, commonly referred to as sugar diabetes, in which the pancreas does not produce enough insulin to control glucose (sugar) levels.

diuretic—a drug that reduces excess fluid in the body by increasing the amount of urine excreted.

edema—a swollen area resulting from abnormal accumulation of fluid.

elixir—a palatable solution used as an accessory substance for a drug; may contain alcohol.

emetic—a substance that induces vomiting.

endocrine—pertaining to glands that produce hormones.

endocrine disorders—any conditions that alter the body's delicate hormone balance, such as menstrual changes or breast enlargement.

euphoria—an exaggerated state of well being.

expectorant—a substance that reduces accumulations of phlegm and mucus in the respiratory tract by aiding its expulsion by inducing coughing.

flatulence—gas in the digestive system.

generic—the standard name of a drug that may be produced by more than one manufacturer under more than one registered brand name.

germicidal—an agent capable of killing microorganisms ("germs").

heart disorders—any condition causing the heart to function less effectively, such as a change in the heart's rhythm.

histamine—a substance released in the body, in response to exposure to an allergen, that causes inflammation and congestion.

hyperglycemia—excessive glucose in the blood.

hypersensitivity—extreme response to a drug so that even a small amount may be intolerable.

hypertension—prolonged high blood pressure.

hypnotic—a substance causing sedation or sleep.

hypoglycemia—abnormally low glucose in the blood.

hypotension—low blood pressure.

infection—a disease caused by microorganisms.

inflammation—swelling, pain, reddening, heat, or other tissue changes due to injury or infection.

interferon—a protein produced by the body that helps protect against invasions of infectious or irritating substances.

jaundice—a condition caused by liver and gall bladder dysfunction that is characterized by yellow-tinged eyes and skin.

kidney disorders—disorders of the kidneys, such as infection or stones, which can cause: fluid retention; distended abdomen; pain and tenderness in the back, lower abdomen, and groin; frequent, urgent, painful, and burning urination; blood and pus in the urine; and scanty urine output.

laxative—an agent that helps evacuate the bowels.

liver disorders—disorders of the liver, such as infection (hepatitis) and scarring (cirrhosis), which can cause: dark urine, light stools, yellow tinged skin and eyes (jaundice), distention of the abdomen, and enlargement and tenderness of the liver under the right ribs.

MAO inhibitor (monoamine oxidase inhibitor)—a type of antidepressant drug.

musculo-skeletal—pertaining to muscles and bones.

narcotic—any substance used for pain relief with effects similar to morphine.

palpitation—a throbbing chest sensation caused by a rapid or irregular heartbeat.

peptic ulcer—an erosion in the lining of the stomach or duodenum.

phlebitis—an inflamed vein, often occurring in the leg.

photosensitivity—exaggerated reaction of skin to light or sun rays; may be caused by drugs, cosmetics, or certain diseases.

psychomotor—pertaining to emotional and physical activity.

psychosis—a mental disorder in which the capacity to communicate, recognize reality, and relate to others is impaired enough to interfere with the ordinary demands of life.

pulmonary—relating to the lungs.

regimen—a therapeutic program or course of action.

renal—relating to the kidneys.

sedative—a drug that produces a calming or relaxing effect.

side effect—an undesired response to a drug that is not the intended therapeutic effect.

stimulant—a substance that increases mental or physical activity.

stroke—a condition resulting from a hemorrhage or a clot in a blood vessel, particularly in the brain.

superinfection—a secondary infection superimposed on the initial infection and not susceptible to the drugs used to treat the original infection.

suspension—a substance that requires mixing prior to use to disperse undissolved particles.

symptom—a change in the body's function, sensation, or appearance that indicates an illness.

syndrome—several symptoms that collectively indicate a specific illness.

systemic—pertaining to the entire body.

topical—pertaining to a surface area of the body.

tranquilizer—a drug that produces a calming effect without inducing sleep.

urinary difficulties—dysfunction of the urinary system with such symptoms as: incontinence, frequency, urgency, or painful urination.

urogenital—relating to the organs of the genital and urinary systems.

vaccine—a preparation that stimulates the body's defenses and reduces susceptibility to infection from certain viruses or bacteria.

vascular system—vessels, such as arteries, veins, and capillaries, that convey blood and fluids.

venereal—pertaining to sexual intercourse and infections transmitted by it.

vertigo—dizziness; the sensation that one's surroundings are spinning.

PRESCRIPTION AND NONPRESCRIPTION DRUGS

The prescription and nonprescription drugs that follow are grouped by disease category. Below are some general guidelines that should be observed when taking *any* drug.

HOW TO USE DRUGS EFFECTIVELY AND SAFELY

Tell your doctor:
- if you are pregnant, breast-feeding, or planning to become pregnant
- if you are allergic by nature or have had previous allergic or adverse reactions to any drug
- *all* medicines you are currently taking
- what recommended drugs you are *not* taking according to your doctor's instructions

Learn from your doctor:
- the drug's generic name, dosage, and purpose
- how and when to take the medicine; when to discontinue it
- any special precautions, particularly regarding any restrictions of activity, or of foods, beverages, or other medicines
- if the prescription can be refilled, how, and how often

Call your doctor immediately if:
- you are concerned that the medicine is causing a problem
- your response to the drug is severe or not as predicted
- you have developed itching, skin rash, hives, breathing problems, or swelling of the face (possible allergic reactions)

Do not:
- share medicines (give or take someone else's for a "similar" problem)
- alter the recommended dosage or frequency
- pressure your doctor to give you a drug
- take more medicine than necessary
- take medicines in the dark (for example, those on your bedside table) because you may take the wrong one

Storage:
- Keep all medicine in labeled bottles and do not remove labels
- Flush discontinued medicine down the toilet
- Refrigerate medicine only when so instructed
- Keep medicine (and all potentially toxic substances) away from children
- Store medicine in a cool, dry, dark cupboard (not a hot and steamy bathroom cupboard), unless instructed otherwise
- Keep a standard "teaspoon" in the medicine cabinet

Children:
- Do not give a child under one year old any drug without a doctor's recommendation
- Adjust dosages according to child's age and body weight following your doctor's advice

Pharmacist:
- If possible, use the same pharmacist for all your prescriptions
- Become acquainted with your pharmacist

Drug Record:
- As provided in designated areas in this book, keep a record of drugs (and vaccines) you have taken or are taking, and record your allergic or adverse reactions to these drugs along with your personal experience of the drug's therapeutic and side effects
- Relate the information on your drug record when changing doctors or pharmacists

Allergies

The body has a defense system to protect itself against infectious or irritating agents. This immune system is in part made up of "antibodies" in the blood, which surround and remove the unwanted substances. When this event occurs, some pain, swelling, and redness may occur, for example, as in a sore throat. For many different reasons, some people have a more active defense system than others and a greater sensitivity to certain irritants, such as dust or pollen. In these individuals, medicines can help reduce the swelling, tightness or congestion, which occur when their immune systems overreact and histamines are released. Antihistamines and decongestants are commonly used to decrease the effects of the overreaction; hormones (corticosteroids) are occasionally used to "turn off" the immune system itself; and mild tranquilizers are sometimes prescribed to reduce the anxiety that contributed to or resulted from the allergic reaction.

PRESCRIPTION DRUGS

Brompheniramine maleate ☐C☐ ☐I☐
Brand: Dimetane Extentabs (Robins)
Tablet
Indication: allergy
Action: reduces congestion and inflammation (antihistamine)
Possible side effects: anorexia; nausea; vomiting; diarrhea; constipation; dry mouth, nose, and throat; fatigue; sedation; confusion; diminished coordination; blurred vision; irritability; ringing in ears; *photosensitivity; *palpitations; *urinary difficulties; *blood disorders; rash and other allergic reactions*

Brompheniramine maleate, guaifenesin, phenylephrine hydrochloride, phenylpropanolamine hydrochloride. See *Ear, Nose, and Throat*

Brompheniramine maleate, guaifenesin, phenylephrine hydrochloride, phenylpropanolamine hydrochloride, codeine phosphate. See *Ear, Nose, and Throat*

Brompheniramine maleate, phenylephrine hydrochloride, phenylpropanolamine hydrochloride. See *Ear, Nose, and Throat*

Caramiphen edisylate, chlorpheniramine maleate, phenylpropanolamine hydrochloride, isopropamide iodide. See *Respiratory System*

Chlorpheniramine maleate ☐C☐ ☐I☐
Brand: Chlor-Trimeton Repetabs (Schering)
Tablet
Indication: allergy
Action: reduces congestion and inflammation (antihistamine)
Possible side effects: anorexia; nausea; vomiting; diarrhea; constipation; dry mouth, nose, and throat; fatigue; sedation; confusion; diminished coordination; blurred vision; irritability; ringing in ears; *photosensitivity; *palpitations; *urinary difficulties; *blood disorders; rash and other allergic reactions*

Chlorpheniramine maleate, phenylpropanolamine hydrochloride, isopropamide iodide. See *Ear, Nose, and*

Throat

Codeine phosphate, guaifenesin, pseudoephedrine hydrochloride, triprolidine hydrochloride. See *Respiratory System*

Codeine sulfate, bromodiphenhydramine hydrochloride, diphenhydramine hydrochloride, ammonium chloride, potassium guaiacolsulfonate. See *Ear, Nose, and Throat*

Cyproheptadine hydrochloride ☐I☐

Brand: Periactin (Merck Sharp & Dohme)

Tablet, Liquid

Indications: allergy; sinus headache

Action: reduces congestion and inflammation (antihistamine)

Possible side effects: anorexia; nausea; vomiting; diarrhea; constipation; dry mouth, nose, and throat; fatigue; sedation; confusion; diminished coordination; blurred vision; irritability; ringing in ears; *photosensitivity; palpitations; *urinary difficulties; *blood disorders; rash and other allergic reactions*

Dexamethasone. See *Musculo-Skeletal System*

Dexbrompheniramine maleate, pseudoephedrine sulfate. See *Ear, Nose, and Throat*

Dexchlorpheniramine maleate ☐C☐ ☐I☐

Brand: Polaramine Tabs (Schering)

Tablet

Indication: allergy

Action: reduces congestion and inflammation (antihistamine)

Possible side effects: anorexia; nausea; vomiting; diarrhea; constipation; dry mouth, nose, and throat; fatigue; sedation; confusion; diminished coordination; blurred vision; irritability; ringing in ears; *photosensitivity; palpitations; *urinary difficulties; *blood disorders; rash and other allergic reactions*

Diphenhydramine hydrochloride ☐C☐ ☐F☐ ☐I☐

Brand: Benadryl, Benylin Cough Syrup (Parke-Davis)

Tablet, Capsule, Liquid, Injection

Indications: allergy; motion sickness; Parkinsonism

Actions: reduces congestion and inflammation (antihistamine); reduces symptoms of Parkinsonism

Possible side effects: anorexia; nausea; vomiting; diarrhea; constipation; dry mouth, nose, and throat; fatigue; sedation; confusion; diminished coordination; blurred vision; irritability; ringing in ears; *photosensitivity; palpitations; *urinary difficulties; *blood disorders; rash and other allergic reactions*

Epinephrine hydrochloride ☐I☐

Generic manufacturers: Abbott; Smith, Miller and Patch

Liquid, Injection

Indications: allergy; asthma; bronchial spasm

Actions: reduces congestion and inflammation (antihistamine); relaxes bronchial muscles

Possible side effects: nausea; vomiting; dry mouth; restlessness; tremors; headache; cold hands and feet; increased perspiring; *palpitations; high blood pressure; rash and other allergic reactions*

Hydroxyzine hydrochloride. See *Central Nervous System*

Phenylpropanolamine hydrochloride, phenylephrine hydrochloride, phenyltoloxamine citrate, chlorpheniramine maleate. See *Ear, Nose, and Throat*

Allergies

Type of Allergy	Symptom	Common Allergens	Possible Treatment
Hay Fever	sneezing, eye irritation, cough, runny nose (seasonal)	pollens, molds, dust	avoidance of allergen, desensitization, antihistamines
Allergic Rhinitis	sneezing, eye irritation, cough, runny nose (year round)	pollens, molds, dust, animal danders, feathers	avoidance of allergen, antihistamines, vasoconstrictors, desensitization
Bronchial Asthma	breathing difficulty, wheezing, cough, tightness in chest	pollens, molds, dust, animal danders, infection, insecticides, foods, cosmetics, drugs, feathers	avoidance of allergen, bronchodilators, corticosteroids
Eczema	itching, swelling, blisters, scaling, rash	foods, drugs, pollens, dust, spores, cosmetics, chemicals, fabrics, detergents	avoidance of allergen, antihistamines, corticosteroids
Hives	rash, welts, itching	stress, foods, drugs, pollen, dust, spores, cosmetics, chemicals, fabrics	avoidance of allergen, antihistamines, corticosteroids
Contact Dermatitis	rash, itching	plants (poison ivy, oak, and sumac), cosmetics, detergents, chemicals, metals, fabrics, drugs	avoidance of allergen, antihistamines, corticosteroids, topical antipruritic
Drug Allergy	rash, welts, fever, nausea, headache, fatigue, itching, breathing difficulty, wheezing	antibiotics (especially penicillin), insulin, sedatives, tranquilizers, anticonvulsants, topical creams and ointments	avoidance of allergen, antihistamines, corticosteroids
Food Allergy	itching, nausea, vomiting, diarrhea, cramps, constipation, rash, welts, tingling of lips or tongue	milk, eggs, nuts, chocolate, shellfish, fish, grains, fruits, vegetables, meats, fowl	avoidance of allergen, antihistamines
Insect Venom	itching, breathing difficulty, nausea, cramps, dizziness	bees, hornets, wasps, yellowjackets	desensitization, immunization, antihistamines, corticosteroids, epinephrine
Conjunctivitis	eye itching, watering, swelling, redness	pollens, molds, dust, animal danders, drugs, cosmetics, chlorine, infection	antihistamines, corticosteroids
Anaphylactic Reaction	rash, breathing difficulty, swelling of face and throat, fever, swollen joints, shock, death	drugs, insect venom	emergency medical treatment, such as adrenalin or corticosteroids

Prednisolone acetate, sulfacetamide sodium. See *Eyes*

Prednisolone sodium phosphate. See *Eyes*

Prednisolone sodium phosphate, sulfacetamide sodium.
See *Eyes*

Promethazine hydrochloride, potassium guaiacolsulfonate.
See *Ear, Nose, and Throat*

**Promethazine hydrochloride, potassium guaiacolsulfonate,
codeine phosphate.** See *Ear, Nose, and Throat*

**Promethazine hydrochloride, potassium guaiacolsulfonate,
phenylephrine hydrochloride.** See *Ear, Nose, and
Throat*

**Promethazine hydrochloride, potassium guaiacolsulfonate,
phenylephrine hydrochloride, codeine phosphate.** See
Ear, Nose, and Throat

**Pseudoephedrine hydrochloride, triprolidine hydro-
chloride.** See *Ear, Nose, and Throat*

Triamcinolone. See *Musculo-Skeletal System*

Tripelennamine hydrochloride, ephedrine sulfate   ☐

Brand: PBZ (Geigy)

Tablet

Indications: allergic nasal congestion; conjunctivitis; hay
fever; skin rash; hives

Action: reduces congestion and inflammation (antihistamine)

Possible side effects: anorexia; nausea; vomiting; diarrhea;
constipation; dry mouth, nose, and throat; fatigue; sedation; confusion; diminished coordination; blurred vision;
irritability; ringing in ears; *photosensitivity; *palpitations; *urinary difficulties; *blood disorders; rash and
other allergic reactions*

NONPRESCRIPTION DRUGS

Alka-Seltzer Plus. See *Respiratory System*

Allerest (Pharmacraft)

Tablet, Capsule

Indications: hay fever; allergy; cold; congestion

Action: reduces congestion and inflammation (antihistamine)

A.R.M. Allergy Relief Medicine (Menley & James)

Tablet

Indications: allergy; nasal and sinus congestion

Action: reduces congestion and inflammation (antihistamine)

Chlor-Trimeton (Schering)

Tablet, Liquid

Indications: hay fever; sinus congestion; allergy

Action: reduces congestion and inflammation (antihistamine)

Chlor-Trimeton Decongestant. See *Respiratory System*

Coricidin Sinus Headache Tablets (Extra Strength). See
Ear, Nose, and Throat

Dimetane (Robins)

Tablet, Liquid

Indication: hay fever; allergy

Action: reduces congestion and inflammation (antihistamine)

Dristan. See *Respiratory System*

4-Way Long Acting Nasal Spray. See *Respiratory System*

Neo-Synephrine. See *Respiratory System*

Novahistine (Dow)

Liquid, Tablet

Indication: sinus or nasal congestion of hay fever, cold, or
sinusitis

Action: reduces congestion and inflammation (antihistamine)

Novahistine DMX. See *Respiratory System*

Novahistine Sinus Tablets (Dow)
Tablet
Indications: congestion; irritated eyes and nose; headache; pain of cold, sinusitis, flu, allergy, or viral infection
Action: reduces congestion and inflammation (antihistamine)
Nyquil Nighttime Colds Medicine. See *Respiratory System*
Primatene. See *Respiratory System*
Rhinosyn DM, Rhinosyn-X. See *Respiratory System*
Rhinosyn Syrup, Rhinosyn-PD. See *Ear, Nose, and Throat*
Sinarest Tablets (Pharmacraft)
Tablet
Indications: hay fever; cold; sinusitis
Action: reduces congestion and inflammation (antihistamine)
Sine-Off AF Aspirin-Free Extra Strength Tablets (Menley & James)
Tablet
Indications: allergic sinusitis; sinusitis; cold
Actions: relieves pain; reduces congestion and postnasal drip
Sine-Off Once-A-Day Sinus Spray. See *Respiratory System*
Sine-Off Tablets-Aspirin Formula (Menley & James)
Tablet
Indications: allergic sinusitis; cold
Actions: relieves pain; reduces congestion and postnasal drip
Sinutab Extra Strength (Warner-Lambert)
Tablet, Capsule
Indications: hay fever; sinus headache and congestion
Action: reduces congestion and inflammation (antihistamine)
Sinutab-II Tablets. See *Ear, Nose, and Throat*
Sominex. See *Nervous System*
Symptom 3 (Parke-Davis)
Liquid
Indication: hay fever
Action: reduces congestion and inflammation (antihistamine)
Teldrin (Smith Kline & French)
Capsule
Indication: allergy
Action: reduces congestion and inflammation (antihistamine)
Triaminicin Tablets (Dorsey)
Tablet
Indications: hay fever; allergy; cold
Action: reduces congestion and inflammation (antihistamine)
Triaminic Syrup (Dorsey)
Liquid
Indications: allergy; cold; sinusitis
Action: reduces congestion and inflammation (antihistamine)
Unisom. See *Nervous System*
Vicks Sinex Long-Acting Decongestant Nasal Spray (Vicks)
Spray
Indications: hay fever; allergy; sinusitis; cold
Action: reduces congestion and inflammation (antihistamine)

Cancer

Cancer is a disease in which the normal production of new cells goes out of control. As a result, the cells can rapidly multiply, form clumps or masses (tumors), and spread through the bloodstream to form masses in other parts of the body (metastases). Although many people believe that the presence of cancer means imminent death, this is usually not the case. Most people live a significant length of time after being diagnosed as having cancer, and increasingly larger numbers of people are cured. Treatments include the surgical removal of the cancerous mass, radiation therapy to destroy the multiplying cells, and different kinds of drug therapy.

Most cancer drugs work by slowing down the uncontrolled growth of cells. Unfortunately, many of these drugs not only affect the growth of cancer cells but also decrease the growth of normal cells. The normal cells most commonly affected by these cancer drugs are cells that the body is continually producing at a rapid rate, such as skin and blood cells. For this reason, the doctor must adjust the cancer drugs so that they limit the growth of the cancer cells but do not limit too severely the growth of normal cells. For instance, if the numbers of blood cells are reduced, the individual may become anemic or increasingly susceptible to infections, or may tend to bleed easily. Finally, the side effects of cancer drugs tend to be more severe than the side effects from other drugs, but this discomfort is usually acceptable if the patient and doctor believe that the cancer drugs will be effective.

PRESCRIPTION DRUGS

Asparaginase
Brand: Elspar (Merck Sharp & Dohme)
Injection
Indication: leukemia
Action: decreases cancer growth by interfering with cell division
Possible side effects: anorexia; nausea; vomiting; abdominal cramps; weight loss; sleepiness; fatigue; headache; irritability; confusion; agitation; hallucinations; depression; decrease in blood sugar level; chills; *high fever; inflammation of pancreas; *blood disorders; *liver disorders; kidney failure; coma; rash and other allergic reactions*

Betamethasone
Brand: Celestone (Schering)
Tablet, Liquid, Cream
Indications: cancer; glandular, rheumatic, and blood disorders; skin, eye, respiratory, and gastrointestinal diseases; allergic states.
Actions: decreases inflammation; modifies immune responses
Possible side effects: fluid and electrolyte disturbances; abdominal pain; headache; dizziness; muscle weakness; increased sweating; change in sugar metabolism; menstrual changes; *delayed wound healing; suppression of growth in children; cataracts; glaucoma; ulcer perforation; bone softening and fractures*

Carmustine (BCNU)
Brand: BiCNU (Bristol)
Injection
Indication: a variety of cancers
Action: decreases tumor growth by interfering with chemical process inside cell
Possible side effects: nausea; vomiting; *liver disorders; *bone marrow depression*

Chlorambucil
Brand: Leukeran (Burroughs Wellcome)
Tablet

Indication: a variety of cancers

Action: decreases tumor growth by interfering with cell division

Possible side effects: nausea; vomiting; *bone marrow depression; severe *blood disorders*

Chlorotrianisene. See *Hormones*

Cisplatin

Brand: Platinol (Bristol)

Injection

Indication: cancer of testes and ovaries

Action: decreases cancer growth by interfering with cell division

Possible side effects: anorexia; nausea; vomiting; low blood pressure; ringing in ears; facial swelling; hearing loss; wheezing; *irregular heartbeat; loss of taste; seizures; *kidney disorders; *bone marrow depression*

Conjugated estrogen. See *Hormones*

Dacarbazine

Brand: DTIC-Dome (Dome)

Injection

Indication: skin cancer

Action: decreases cancer growth by interfering with cell division

Possible side effects: anorexia; nausea; vomiting; malaise; *photosensitivity; loss of hair; muscle pain; fever; *bone marrow depression; *liver or *kidney disorders; severe *blood disorders; rash and other allergic reactions*

Dactinomycin

Brand: Cosmegen (Merck Sharp & Dohme)

Injection

Indication: a variety of cancers

Action: decreases tumor growth

Possible side effects: anorexia; nausea; vomiting; diarrhea; fatigue; muscle pain; changes in skin color; loss of hair; inflammation; anemia; *bone marrow depression; high blood pressure with bleeding into the tissues; rash and other allergic reactions*

Dexamethasone. See *Musculo-Skeletal System*

Diethylstilbestrol. See *Hormones*

Diethylstilbestrol diphosphate

Brand: Stilphostrol (Dome)

Tablet, Injection

Indication: cancer of prostate

Action: decreases prostatic cancer by increasing estrogens

Possible side effects: anorexia; nausea; vomiting; abdominal cramps; bloating; fatigue; dizziness; headache; nervousness; irritability; swelling; fluid retention; weight gain or loss; pain at site of injection; breast tenderness and enlargement; loss of hair; backache; jaundice; decreased libido; high blood pressure; itching; *blood clots; rash and other allergic reactions*

Doxorubicin hydrochloride

Brand: Adriamycin (Adria)

Injection

Indication: a variety of cancers

Action: decreases tumor growth

Possible side effects: anorexia; nausea; vomiting; diarrhea; flushing; chills; fever; loss of hair; red urine; inflammation of mouth; aggravation of gout; ulceration; *liver disorders; congestive heart failure; rash and other allergic reactions*

Dromostanolone propionate

Brand: Drolban (Lilly)

Injection

Indication: breast cancer

Action: affects hormone-dependent tumors by altering hormone levels

Possible side effects: masculinization; fluid retention; increased calcium blood levels

Ethinyl estradiol. See *Hormones*

Floxuridine

Brand: FUDR (Roche)

Injection

Indication: cancers of the gastrointestinal tract and liver

Action: decreases tumor growth by interfering with chemical process inside cell

Possible side effects: anorexia; nausea; vomiting; diarrhea; weakness; loss of hair; fever; redness of skin; inflammation of mouth and intestines; ulcers; **bone marrow depression; rash and other allergic reactions*

Fluorouracil

Brand: Adrucil Injectable (Adria)

Injection

Indication: a variety of cancers

Action: decreases tumor growth by interfering with chemical process inside cell

Possible side effects: anorexia; nausea; vomiting; diarrhea; euphoria; nosebleeds; *photosensitivity; sensitivity of the eyes to light; loss of hair or nails; **liver disorders; *bone marrow depression; heart failure; rash and other allergic reactions*

Fluorouracil

Brand: Efudex (Roche)

Liquid (topical), Cream

Indication: cancers of the skin

Action: decreases tumor growth by interfering with chemical process inside the cell

Possible side effects: insomnia; pain; burning at application site; inflammation of mouth; *photosensitivity; *rash and other allergic reactions*

Liothyronine sodium. See *Hormones*

Lomustine (CCNU)

Brand: CeeNU (Bristol)

Capsule

Indications: brain tumor; Hodgkin's disease

Action: decreases tumor growth by interfering with chemical process inside the cell and cell division

Possible side effects: anorexia; nausea; vomiting; diarrhea; loss of hair; **bone marrow depression*

Mechlorethamine hydrochloride

Brand: Mustargen (Merck Sharp & Dohme)

Injection

Indication: a variety of cancers

Action: decreases tumor growth by interfering with cell division

Possible side effects: anorexia; nausea; vomiting; diarrhea; weakness; susceptibility to infection; impaired reproductive capability; *blood clots*

Melphalan

Brand: Alkeran (Burroughs Wellcome)

Tablet

Indication: cancer of the bone marrow

Action: decreases cancer growth by interfering with cell division

Possible side effects: nausea; vomiting; diarrhea; loss of hair; mouth ulcers; *bone marrow depression; bleeding from the gut*

Mercaptopurine

Brand: Purinethol (Burroughs Wellcome)

Tablet

Indication: certain types of leukemia

Action: decreases cancer growth by interfering with chemical process inside the cell

Possible side effects: anorexia; nausea; vomiting; diarrhea; fever; jaundice; *bone marrow depression; *kidney and *liver disorders*

Methotrexate

Generic manufacturer: Lederle

Tablet, Injection

Indications: a variety of cancers

Action: decreases tumor growth by interfering with chemical process inside the cell

Possible side effects: anorexia; nausea; vomiting; diarrhea; fatigue; blurred vision; chills; fever; decrease in white blood cells; *liver disorders; *bone marrow depression; kidney failure; rash and other allergic reactions*

Methyltestosterone. See *Hormones*

Mithramycin

Brand: Mithracin (Dome)

Injection

Indication: cancer of the testis

Action: decreases tumor growth by interfering with chemical process inside the cell

Possible side effects: anorexia; nausea; vomiting; diarrhea; drowsiness; fatigue; headache; depression; inflammation of mouth; fever; decrease in blood clotting; *bone marrow depression, especially with nosebleeds; *liver and *kidney disorders; rash and other allergic reactions*

Mitomycin

Brand: Mutamycin (Bristol)

Injection

Indication: cancer of the stomach or pancreas

Action: decreases tumor growth by interfering with chemical process inside the cell

Possible side effects: anorexia; nausea; vomiting; diarrhea; fatigue; blurred vision; headache; pain at site of injection; fever; *bone marrow depression; *kidney and lung disorders*

Mitotane

Brand: Lysodren (Bristol)

Tablet

Indication: adrenal cortical cancer

Action: decreases cancer growth by inhibiting production of adrenal cortex hormones

Possible side effects: anorexia; nausea; vomiting; diarrhea; lethargy; sleepiness; *rash and other allergic reactions*

Tamoxifen citrate

Brand: Nolvadex (Stuart)

Tablet

Indication: breast cancer in postmenopausal women

Action: affects hormone-dependent tumors by altering hormone level

Possible side effects: nausea; vomiting; hot flashes; vaginal bleeding and discharge

Testolactone
Brand: Teslac (Squibb)
Tablet, Injection
Indication: breast cancer
Action: decreases breast cancer growth (in women only)
Possible side effects: anorexia; nausea; vomiting; aches; pain at site of injection; swelling of extremities; high blood pressure

Vinblastine sulfate
Brand: Velban (Lilly)
Injection
Indication: a variety of cancers
Action: decreases tumor growth
Possible side effects: anorexia; nausea; vomiting; diarrhea; constipation; difficult bowel movements; abdominal pain; weakness; dizziness; headache; numbness; loss of hair; rectal bleeding; depression; inflammation of nerves; inflammation of pharynx; *bleeding of peptic ulcer; loss of deep-tendon reflexes; convulsions*

Vincristine sulfate
Brand: Oncovin (Lilly)
Injection
Indication: a variety of cancers
Action: decreases cancer growth by interfering with cell division
Possible side effects: constipation; loss of hair; inflammation of nerves; sensory loss; decrease in white blood cells; walking difficulties; *muscle wasting*

Cardiovascular System

Heart Disease

The function of the heart is to pump oxygen-carrying blood from the lungs to cells throughout the body. If the heart suddenly stops pumping, the brain and all other organs die from lack of oxygen. If the heart does not stop but only fails to pump adequately ("heart failure"), the body's organs suffer the consequences; for example, the individual may feel lightheaded from insufficient oxygen to the brain or may feel fatigue and cramps with exertion from insufficient oxygen to the muscles. Furthermore, because a "backup" occurs in the pumping system, the lungs, liver, legs, and other tissues become congested with fluid ("congestive heart failure"). This congestion can cause edema and shortness of breath, particularly when exercising or lying flat without pillows.

To treat heart failure, medications can be used to help the heart pump more effectively (see chart). **Digitalis preparations** increase the strength of heart muscle. **Anti-arrhythmic agents** adjust the rhythm of the heart to help it beat more regularly and therefore efficiently. **Diuretics** ("water pills") help remove some of the excess fluid. **Hypotensive drugs** lower the blood pressure so the heart does not have to force the oxygenated blood through narrowed blood vessels. **Vasodilators** open the constricted blood vessels. **Antilipimic drugs** help prevent the blood vessels from becoming too clogged with deposits of fat.

In addition, along with other tissues not receiving sufficient oxygen, heart failure may decrease the amount of oxygen to the heart muscles. If this decrease is sudden and severe, a portion of the heart muscle may die and cause the pump to become impaired ("heart attack"). When the decrease in oxygen to the heart muscles is temporary and related to demands for the heart to work harder (for example, going upstairs or shoveling snow), the cramped heart muscles cause a particular kind of pain sensation ("angina pectoris"), which may be a pressing on the chest, a tingling down the left arm, a tightness in the throat, a gnawing in the stomach or back, or an ache in the jaw. **Nitroglycerine** can help relieve this sensation along with the already-mentioned ways to make the heart pump more effectively.

A doctor should always be consulted to determine the cause of the heart failure. Possible causes include clogged blood vessels to the heart muscles (from coronary artery disease), impaired valves inside the heart (from birth defects or rheumatic heart disease), irregular heart rhythm (from poor circulation to the heart's conduction system), high blood pressure, kidney trouble, anemia, and so on. The treatment will depend on the cause.

Hypertension

Blood pressure is the force of the blood on the walls of the body's larger arteries. In general, if these blood vessels are narrow (constricted), the force on the walls of the vessels will be greater. This greater force can cause pounding headaches and can eventually lead to a break in the blood vessels; for example, a hemorrhage ("stroke") in the brain. Furthermore, the constricted blood vessels make it more difficult for certain organs to function: muscles receive less oxygen and cramp; the kidneys cannot filter as well and this can lead to swelling; and the heart muscles may receive less oxygen through the narrowed vessels and pump less effectively. High blood pressure has many causes, including certain internal hormonal problems of the kidneys. Treatment will be based on the underlying cause. Furthermore, because the treatment may continue for many years as adjustments and changes in medication occur, a good working relationship with the doctor is necessary. The patient must be able to ask about annoying side effects and to talk honestly about whether the drugs are actually being taken as prescribed.

PRESCRIPTION DRUGS

Acetazolamide $\boxed{\text{P}}$
Brand: Diamox (Lederle)
Tablet, Capsule
Indications: fluid retention; glaucoma; epilepsy
Action: reduces fluid retention
Possible side effects: urinary frequency; anorexia; nausea; vomiting; diarrhea; constipation; dizziness; drowsiness; nearsightedness; aggravation of diabetes; *confusion; depression; tingling sensations; muscle spasm; *kidney and *liver disorders; convulsions; rash and other allergic reactions*

Chlorothiazide $\boxed{\text{P}}$
Brand: Diuril (Merck Sharp & Dohme)
Tablet

Indications: fluid retention; hypertension
Actions: reduces fluid retention; lowers blood pressure
Possible side effects: urinary frequency; indigestion; anorexia; nausea; vomiting; diarrhea; constipation; lightheadedness when arising from prone position; dizziness; headache; fatigue; aggravation of diabetes or gout; *decrease in potassium level with muscle weakness and cramps; yellow or blurred vision; hepatitis with jaundice; inflammation of pancreas with severe abdominal pain; *bone marrow depression with fever, unusual bleeding or bruising, and sore throat; rash and other allergic reactions*

Chlorothiazide, reserpine ☐ I ☐ P
Brand: Diupres (Merck Sharp & Dohme)
Tablet
Indication: hypertension
Actions: lowers blood pressure; reduces fluid retention; tranquilizes
Possible side effects: anorexia; nausea; indigestion; vomiting; diarrhea; constipation; urinary frequency; sedation; drowsiness; lethargy; weakness; lightheadedness when arising from prone position; dizziness; headache; depression; fatigue; insomnia or nightmares; agitation; nervousness; dry mouth; weight gain; flushing; impotence; fluid retention; nasal congestion; blurred vision; breast enlargement; menstrual changes; aggravation of ulcers, glaucoma, diabetes, or gout; *decrease in potassium level with muscle weakness and cramps; irregular heartbeat; yellow or blurred vision; hepatitis with jaundice; confusion; inflammation of pancreas with severe abdominal pain; hallucinations; *bone marrow depression with fever, unusual bleeding or bruising, and sore*

Cardiovascular Problems

Symptoms	Possible Cause	Possible Treatments
lightheadedness muscle cramps leg swelling shortness of breath (particularly with exercise)	congestive heart failure	strengthen heart muscles (digitalis preparations)
		adjust heart rhythm (anti-arrythmic agents)
		remove excess fluid (diuretics)
		lower blood pressure (hypotensives)
		widen blood vessels (vasodilators)
		decrease clogged vessels (antilipemic drugs)
pressing chest pain ("angina")	cramped heart muscles	nitroglycerine
headaches dizziness leg swelling strokes heart attacks	high blood pressure	hypotensives

throat; rash and other allergic reactions

See also listings for Chlorothiazide and Reserpine

Note: avoid highly spiced foods and carbonated beverages

Chlorthalidone [F] [P]

Brand: Hygroton (USV)

Tablet

Indication: hypertension

Actions: lowers blood pressure; reduces fluid retention

Possible side effects: anorexia; nausea; vomiting; diarrhea; constipation; urinary frequency; headache; dizziness; vertigo; aggravation of diabetes and gout; impotence; *decrease in potassium level with muscle spasm, cramps, or weakness; jaundice; rash and other allergic reactions*

Chlorthalidone, reserpine [F] [P]

Brand: Regroton (USV)

Tablet

Indication: hypertension

Actions: lowers blood pressure; reduces fluid retention

Possible side effects: urinary frequency; anorexia; nausea; vomiting; diarrhea; constipation; sedation; lethargy; weakness; headache; dizziness; vertigo; depression; insomnia or nightmares; agitation; nervousness; dry mouth; weight gain; flushing; aggravation of diabetes and gout; impotence; fluid retention; nasal congestion; blurred vision; breast enlargement; menstrual changes; aggravation of ulcers or glaucoma; *decrease in potassium level with muscle spasm, cramps, or weakness; irregular heartbeat; confusion; hallucinations; jaundice; rash and other allergic reactions*

See also listings for Chlorthalidone and Reserpine

Note: avoid highly spiced foods and carbonated beverages

Cholestyramine

Brand: Questran (Mead Johnson)

Powder

Indication: high level of fat in blood

Action: reduces level of fat in blood

Possible side effects: nausea; vomiting; diarrhea; constipation; drowsiness; fatigue; dizziness; headache; backache; increased libido; anxiety; burnt odor to urine; increased urine; *painful urination; muscle, joint, and bone pain; vitamins A, D, and K deficiencies with gradual weakness and weight loss; swollen glands; dental bleeding; anemia; inflammation of eye*

Clofibrate

Brand: Atromid-S (Ayerst)

Capsule

Indication: high level of fat in blood

Action: reduces level of fat in blood

Possible side effects: nausea; vomiting; flatulence; diarrhea; abdominal distress; headache; dizziness; fatigue; flulike symptoms; weight gain; impotence or decreased libido; *cramps or weakness; irregular heartbeat; painful urination; rash and other allergic reactions*

Note: use in conjunction with low fat and carbohydrate diet

Clonidine hydrochloride [I]

Brand: Catapres (Boehringer Ingelheim)

Tablet

Indication: hypertension

Action: lowers blood pressure

Possible side effects: nausea; vomiting; constipation; dry mouth; drowsiness; fatigue; dizziness; headache; insomnia; depression; restlessness; behavioral changes; weight gain or loss; impotence; itching and burning of eyes; *urinary retention; congestive heart failure; rash and other allergic reactions*

Warning: tolerance to this drug develops, requiring frequent reevaluation of treatment

Cyclandelate F

Brand: Cyclospasmol (Ives)

Tablet, Capsule

Indication: circulatory disorders from constriction of blood vessels

Action: dilates blood vessels

Possible side effects: nausea; vomiting; constipation; flushing; headache; weakness; lightheadedness when arising from prone position; *palpitations*

Digitoxin

Generic manufacturer: Purepac

Tablet

Indications: congestive heart failure; irregular heart rhythm

Actions: increases force of muscular contraction; restores normal heart rate and rhythm

Possible side effects: anorexia; nausea; vomiting; diarrhea; breast enlargement; vision disturbances; drowsiness; *abnormal bruising; confusion; rash and other allergic reactions*

Digoxin

Generic manufacturers: Invenex, Purepac

Tablet, Injection

Brands: Lanoxin (Burroughs Wellcome); SK-Digoxin (Smith Kline & French)

Tablet

Indications: congestive heart failure; irregular heart rhythm

Actions: increases force of muscular contraction; restores normal heart rate and rhythm

Possible side effects: anorexia; nausea; vomiting; diarrhea; breast enlargement; vision disturbances; drowsiness; *abnormal bruising; confusion; rash and other allergic reactions*

Dipyridamole

Brand: Persantine (Boehringer Ingelheim)

Tablet

Indication: angina pectoris

Action: dilates heart blood vessels

Possible side effects: nausea; vomiting; constipation; flushing; headache; weakness; lightheadedness when arising from prone position; *palpitations*

Note: take 1 hour before eating; with milk to prevent stomach distress

Disopyramide phosphate

Brand: Norpace (Searle)

Capsule

Indication: heart rhythm disorders

Action: regulates heart rhythm

Possible side effects: anorexia; nausea; vomiting; flatulence; diarrhea; constipation; weight gain; dry mouth; nervousness; dizziness; fatigue; headache; fluid retention; aggravation of diabetes; blurred vision; *jaundice; congestive heart failure and chest pain; rash and other allergic reactions*

Furosemide P

Brand: Lasix Oral (Hoechst-Roussel)
Tablet, Liquid
Indications: hypertension; fluid retention
Actions: lowers blood pressure; reduces fluid retention
Possible side effects: urinary frequency; anorexia; nausea; vomiting; constipation; diarrhea; aggravation of diabetes and gout; dizziness; headache; blurred vision; ringing in ears; *photosensitivity; *decrease in potassium levels with weakness and muscle spasm or cramps; *bone marrow depression*

Guanethidine sulfate
Brand: Ismelin (CIBA)
Tablet
Indication: hypertension
Action: lowers blood pressure
Possible side effects: nausea; vomiting; diarrhea; weight gain; dry mouth; nasal congestion; loss of hair; lightheadedness; depression; dizziness; blurred vision; fluid retention; impotence or impaired ejaculation; *urinary difficulties; muscle aches, tremors, or weakness; *activation of stomach or peptic ulcer; chest pain; rash and other allergic reactions*

Hydralazine hydrochloride
Brand: Apresoline hydrochloride (CIBA)
Tablet
Indication: hypertension
Action: lowers blood pressure
Possible side effects: anorexia; nausea; vomiting; diarrhea; constipation; dizziness; headache; depression; anxiety; fluid retention; flushing; nasal congestion; tremors; cramps; low blood pressure; impotence; *chills and fever; rapid heartbeat; palpitations; irregular heartbeat; hepatitis; *bone marrow depression; chest pain; rash and other allergic reactions*

Hydrochlorothiazide [P]
Generic manufacturers: American Pharmaceutical, Parke-Davis, Premo, Purepac, Rexall
Brands: Esidrix (CIBA), HydroDIURIL (Merck Sharp & Dohme)
Tablet
Indications: fluid retention; hypertension
Actions: reduces fluid retention; lowers blood pressure
Possible side effects: urinary frequency; anorexia; nausea; vomiting; diarrhea; constipation; dizziness; headache; restlessness; aggravation of diabetes or gout; *photosensitivity; *decrease in potassium level with weakness and muscle spasm or cramps; hepatitis with jaundice; *bone marrow depression; rash and other allergic reactions*

Hydrochlorothiazide, reserpine [I] [P]
Brand: Hydropres (Merck Sharp & Dohme)
Tablet
Indication: hypertension
Actions: lowers blood pressure; reduces fluid retention; tranquilizes
Possible side effects: urinary frequency; anorexia; nausea; vomiting; diarrhea; constipation; sedation; lethargy; weakness; dizziness; headache; restlessness; depression; insomnia or nightmares; agitation; nervousness; dry mouth; weight gain; flushing; impotence; fluid retention; nasal congestion; aggravation of diabetes or gout;

*photosensitivity; blurred vision; breast enlargement; menstrual changes; aggravation of ulcers or glaucoma; *irregular heartbeat; confusion; hallucinations; decrease in potassium level with weakness and muscle spasm or cramps; hepatitis with jaundice; *bone marrow depression; rash and other allergic reactions*

See also listings for Hydrochlorothiazide and Reserpine

Note: avoid highly spiced foods and carbonated beverages

Hydroflumethiazide, reserpine   [I]   [P]

Brand: Salutensin (Bristol)

Tablet

Indication: hypertension

Actions: lowers blood pressure; reduces fluid retention; tranquilizes

Possible side effects: urinary frequency; anorexia; nausea; vomiting; diarrhea; constipation; increase in appetite; weight gain; drowsiness; lethargy; sedation; dizziness; headache; vertigo; blurred vision; fluid retention; insomnia; aggravation of diabetes; dry mouth; depression; low blood pressure; impotence; tremors; nasal congestion; flushing; breast enlargement; menstrual changes; agitation; nervousness; aggravation of ulcers or glaucoma; *redness of eye; decrease in white blood cells; anemia; decrease in potassium level with weakness and muscle spasm or cramps; jaundice; irregular heartbeat; confusion; hallucinations; deafness; abnormal bruising; rash and other allergic reactions*

See also listing for Reserpine

Note: avoid highly spiced foods and carbonated beverages

Isosorbide dinitrate

Brands: Isordil (Ives), Sorbitrate (Stuart)

Tablet

Indication: angina pectoris

Action: dilates blood vessels

Possible side effects: nausea; vomiting; constipation; flushing; headache; weakness; lightheadedness when arising from prone position; *palpitations; severe skin rash with skin peeling*

Note: take ½-1 hour before food

Isoxsuprine hydrochloride   [F]

Brand: Vasodilan (Mead Johnson)

Tablet, Injection

Indication: circulatory disorders

Action: dilates blood vessels

Possible side effects: nausea; vomiting; constipation; flushing; headache; weakness; lightheadedness when arising from prone position; *palpitations; severe skin rash with skin peeling*

Methyclothiazide   [P]

Brand: Enduron (Abbott)

Tablet

Indications: hypertension; fluid retention

Actions: lowers blood pressure; reduces fluid retention

Possible side effects: urinary frequency; indigestion; anorexia; nausea; vomiting; diarrhea; constipation; lightheadedness when arising from prone position; dizziness; headache; fatigue; aggravation of diabetes or gout; *decrease in potassium level with muscle weakness and cramps; yellow or blurred vision; hepatitis with jaundice; inflammation of pancreas with severe abdominal pain; *bone marrow depression with fever, unusual* *bleeding or bruising, and sore throat; rash and other allergic reactions*

Methyldopa [I]

Brand: Aldomet (Merck Sharp & Dohme)

Tablet

Indication: hypertension

Action: lowers blood pressure

Possible side effects: nausea; vomiting; diarrhea; constipation; sedation; dizziness; headache; lightheadedness; dry mouth; weight gain; fluid retention; weakness; tremors; nasal congestion; impotence; breast enlargement; fever; depression; *jaundice*

Methyldopa, hydrochlorothiazide [I] [P]

Brand: Aldoril (Merck Sharp & Dohme)

Tablet

Indication: hypertension

Action: lowers blood pressure

Possible side effects: urinary frequency; anorexia; nausea; vomiting; diarrhea; constipation; sedation; dizziness; headache; lightheadedness; restlessness; dry mouth; weight gain; fluid retention; weakness; tremors; nasal congestion; aggravation of diabetes or gout; impotence; *photosensitivity; breast enlargement; fever; depression; decrease in potassium level with weakness and muscle spasm or cramps; hepatitis with jaundice; *bone marrow depression; rash and other allergic reactions*
See also listings for Methyldopa and Hydrochlorothiazide

Metolazone

Brand: Zaroxolyn (Pennwalt)

Tablet

Indications: hypertension; fluid retention

Actions: lowers blood pressure; reduces fluid retention

Possible side effects: urinary frequency; anorexia; nausea; vomiting; diarrhea; constipation; drowsiness; fatigue; dizziness; headache; aggravation of diabetes or gout; *decrease in white blood cells; fainting; irregular heartbeat; decrease in potassium level with weakness and cramps; hepatitis with jaundice; chest pain; rash and other allergic reactions*

Metoprolol tartrate [I]

Brand: Lopressor (Geigy)

Tablet

Indication: hypertension

Action: lowers blood pressure

Possible side effects: diarrhea; fatigue; dizziness; headache; cold hands and feet; insomnia or nightmares; depression; *slow heartbeat; shortness of breath; congestive heart failure*

Niacin

Brands: Nicalex (Merrell-National), Nicobid, Nicolar (Armour), Nico-Span (Key), Nicotinex (Fleming), SK-Niacin (Smith Kline & French)

Tablet, Capsule, Liquid

Indication: high level of fat in blood

Action: reduces level of fat in blood

Possible side effects: nausea; indigestion; vomiting; diarrhea; headache; flushing; tingling; lightheadedness when arising from prone position; feeling of warmth; dry or pigmented skin; dim vision; aggravation of diabetes or gout; *activation of peptic ulcer; hepatitis with jaundice; rash and other allergic reactions*

Nitroglycerin
Generic manufacturers: Lederle, Purepac
Capsule
Brands: Nitro-Bid (Marion), Nitrostat (Parke-Davis)
Capsule, Tablet
Indication: angina pectoris
Action: dilates blood vessels
Possible side effects: nausea; dry mouth; vomiting; dizziness; weakness; flushing; sweating; restlessness; headache; blurred vision; loss of facial color; *palpitations; rash and other allergic reactions*

Papaverine hydrochloride
Brand: Pavabid (Marion)
Capsule
Indication: circulatory disorders
Action: dilates blood vessels
Possible side effects: anorexia; nausea; diarrhea; constipation; abdominal distress; drowsiness; weakness; dizziness; vertigo; headache; flushing; sweating; *rash and other allergic reactions*

Phentolamine
Brand: Regitine (CIBA)
Tablet
Indication: hypertension
Action: lowers blood pressure
Possible side effects: nausea; vomiting; diarrhea; lightheadedness when arising from prone position; weakness; dizziness; flushing; nasal congestion; low blood pressure; *irregular heartbeat*

Potassium chloride   [F]
Generic manufacturers: Invenex, Philips Roxane, Purepac
Brands: Slow-K (CIBA), K-Lyte (Mead Johnson)
Tablet, Liquid, Powder
Indication: potassium deficiency, particularly due to diuretics or severe diarrhea and vomiting
Action: supplements potassium
Possible side effects: nausea; vomiting; abdominal discomfort; diarrhea; low blood pressure; *irregular heartbeat; *kidney disorders; intestinal and gastric ulceration and bleeding; rash and other allergic reactions*
Warning: Do not discontinue abruptly if taking digitalis
Note: avoid potassium-rich diet and salt substitute

Prazosin hydrochloride
Brand: Minipress (Pfizer)
Capsule
Indication: hypertension
Action: lowers blood pressure
Possible side effects: nausea; vomiting; diarrhea; drowsiness; fatigue; dizziness; headache; vertigo; weakness; nervousness; depression; blurred vision; fluid retention; impotence; ringing in ears; dry mouth; nasal congestion; *urinary difficulties; rapid heartbeat; palpitations; fainting; rash and other allergic reactions*

Procainamide hydrochloride
Generic manufacturers: American Pharmaceutical, Lederle, Purepac
Brand: Pronestyl (Squibb)
Capsule, Tablet

Indication: heart rhythm disorders

Action: regulates heart rhythm

Possible side effects: anorexia; nausea; vomiting; diarrhea; weakness; *depression; *bone marrow depression; rash and other allergic reactions*

Propranolol hydrochloride ☐F☐ ☐I☐

Brand: Inderal (Ayerst)

Tablet, Injection

Indications: hypertension; angina pectoris; heart rhythm disorders; migraine headaches

Actions: lowers blood pressure; decreases angina; regulates heart rhythm

Possible side effects: anorexia; nausea; vomiting; diarrhea; constipation; lightheadedness; loss of hair; cold hands and feet; *depression; confusion; hallucinations; *bone marrow depression*

Quinidine sulfate

Generic manufacturers: American Pharmaceutical, Lederle, Lilly, Purepac, Rexall

Tablet, Capsule

Indication: heart rhythm disorders

Action: regulates heart rhythm

Possible side effects: anorexia; nausea; vomiting; diarrhea; lightheadedness; dizziness; flushing; ringing in ears; vision disturbances; agitation; tremors; *confusion; *bone marrow depression; rash and other allergic reactions*

Reserpine ☐I☐

Generic manufacturers: Purepac, Rexall

Tablet

Indication: hypertension

Actions: lowers blood pressure; tranquilizes

Possible side effects: nausea; vomiting; diarrhea; drowsiness; sedation; lethargy; weakness; dizziness; headache; depression; insomnia or nightmares; agitation; nervousness; dry mouth; weight gain; flushing; impotence; fluid retention; nasal congestion; blurred vision; breast enlargement; menstrual changes; aggravation of ulcers or glaucoma; *irregular heartbeat; confusion; hallucinations; rash and other allergic reactions*

Note: avoid highly spiced foods and carbonated beverages

Reserpine, hydralazine hydrochloride, hydrochlorothiazide ☐I☐ ☐P☐

Brand: Ser-Ap-Es (CIBA)

Tablet

Indication: hypertension

Actions: lowers blood pressure; tranquilizes

Possible side effects: urinary frequency; anorexia; nausea; vomiting; diarrhea; constipation; drowsiness; sedation; lethargy; weakness; dizziness; headache; restlessness; depression; anxiety; insomnia or nightmares; agitation; nervousness; weight gain; flushing; impotence; fluid retention; nasal congestion; tremors; cramps; low blood pressure; blurred vision; breast enlargement; menstrual changes; aggravation of diabetes or gout; **photosensitivity; aggravation of ulcers or glaucoma; irregular heartbeat; rapid heartbeat; palpitations; chills and fever; confusion; decrease in potassium level with weakness and muscle spasm or cramps; hepatitis with jaundice; hallucinations; *bone marrow depression; chest pain; rash and other allergic reactions*

See also listings for Reserpine, Hydralazine hydrochloride, and Hydrochlorothiazide

Note: avoid highly spiced foods and carbonated beverages

Spironolactone

Brand: Aldactone (Searle)

Tablet

Indications: fluid retention; kidney disorders; hypertension; potassium deficiency

Actions: increases urination; lowers blood pressure; changes salt balance in kidneys

Possible side effects: nausea; vomiting; diarrhea; indigestion; dry mouth; thirst; dizziness; drowsiness; lethargy; fatigue; headache; weakness; loss of balance; impotence; breast enlargement; (in women) beard growth, deepening of voice, and menstrual changes; *confusion; stomach ulcers and bleeding; rash and other allergic reactions*

Warning: possible *carcinogen

Spironolactone, hydrochlorothiazide P

Brand: Aldactazide (Searle)

Tablet

Indications: fluid retention; congestive heart failure; cirrhosis; kidney disorders; potassium deficiency; hypertension

Actions: reduces fluid retention; lowers blood pressure

Possible side effects: urinary frequency; anorexia; nausea; vomiting; diarrhea; indigestion; constipation; dry mouth; thirst; dizziness; drowsiness; lethargy; fatigue; headache; restlessness; weakness; loss of balance; aggravation of diabetes or gout; *photosensitivity; impotence; breast enlargement; (in women) beard growth, deepening of voice, and menstrual changes; *confusion; decrease in potassium level with weakness and muscle spasm or cramps; stomach ulcers and bleeding; hepatitis with jaundice; *bone marrow depression; rash and other allergic reactions*

See also listing for Spironolactone and Hydrochlorothiazide

Warning: possible *carcinogen

Triamterene, hydrochlorothiazide P

Brand: Dyazide (Smith Kline & French)

Capsule

Indications: hypertension; fluid retention

Actions: lowers blood pressure; lowers fluid retention

Possible side effects: blue urine; urinary frequency; anorexia; nausea; vomiting; diarrhea; constipation; weakness; dizziness; headache; restlessness; *photosensitivity; aggravation of diabetes or gout; abdominal pain; *decrease in potassium level with weakness and muscle spasm or cramps; hepatitis with jaundice; *bone marrow depression; rash and other allergic reactions*

See also listing for Hydrochlorothiazide

Warfarin sodium

Brand: Coumadin (Endo)

Tablet

Indications: blood clots; heart rhythm disorders; coronary heart disease; impaired circulation

Action: slows clotting action of blood

Possible side effects: nausea; vomiting; diarrhea; abnormal bruising; loss of scalp hair; *increased bleeding of nose and gums and appearance of blood in sputum, urine, or stools; fever; rash and other allergic reactions*

Note: avoid Vitamin K

Ear, Nose, and Throat

Because many irritating or infectious substances are carried in the air, the body has an elaborate defensive system built into the upper airway to fight off these potentially harmful agents. However, when this upper respiratory system reacts defensively, the result can be soreness, swelling, congestion, redness, and other signs of inflammation. The medications most commonly used for these symptoms are "antihistamines," which decrease the local reaction of the ear, nose, and throat. Because the infection is often caused by a virus, antibiotics are not prescribed; most antibiotics usually are not effective against these kinds of infectious organisms. Antibiotics may be used when the infection is caused by bacteria, a different type of organism. Often symptoms of the mouth and throat that are caused by the common cold are accompanied by respiratory problems. Many drugs for "upper respiratory" infections will be found in the chapter on the respiratory system.

PRESCRIPTION DRUGS

Brompheniramine maleate. See *Allergies*

Brompheniramine maleate, guaifenesin, phenylephrine hydrochloride, phenylpropanolamine hydrochloride |I|

Brand: Dimetane Expectorant (Robins)

Liquid

Indications: cough; allergy

Actions: suppresses cough; reduces congestion and inflammation (antihistamine); loosens phlegm

Possible side effects: anorexia; nausea; vomiting; diarrhea; constipation; *urinary difficulties; drowsiness; lightheadedness; dry mouth, nose, and throat; blurred vision; nervousness; confusion; headache; insomnia; muscle spasms; *photosensitivity; *irregular heart rhythm with palpitations; *bone marrow depression; rash and other allergic reactions*

Brompheniramine maleate, guaifenesin, phenylephrine hydrochloride, phenylpropanolamine hydrochloride, codeine phosphate |D| |F| |I|

Brand: Dimetane Expectorant-DC (Robins)

Liquid

Indications: cough; allergy

Actions: suppresses cough; reduces congestion and inflammation (antihistamine); loosens phlegm; relieves pain

Possible side effects: anorexia; nausea; vomiting; diarrhea; constipation; *urinary difficulties; drowsiness; lightheadedness; dry mouth, nose, and throat; blurred vision; nervousness; confusion; headache; insomnia; muscle spasms; *photosensitivity; *irregular heart rhythm with palpitations; *bone marrow depression; rash and other allergic reactions*

Brompheniramine maleate, phenylephrine hydrochloride, phenylpropanolamine hydrochloride |I|

Brand: Dimetapp (Robins)

Tablet, Liquid

Indications: upper respiratory congestion; allergy

Action: reduces congestion and inflammation (antihistamine)

Possible side effects: anorexia; nausea; vomiting; diarrhea;

constipation; drowsiness; lightheadedness; dry mouth, nose, and throat; blurred vision; nervousness; confusion; headache; insomnia; *urinary difficulties; muscle spasms; *photosensitivity; *irregular heart rhythm with palpitations; *bone marrow depression; rash and other allergic reactions*

Caramiphen edisylate, chlorpheniramine maleate, phenyl-propanolamine hydrochloride, isopropamide iodide. See *Respiratory System*

Cephalexin. See *Infection*

Chloramphenicol

Brand: Chloromycetin Otic (Parke-Davis)

Liquid (topical)

Indication: superficial infections of external ear canal

Action: treats bacterial infection

*Possible side effects: irritation; burning; itching; swelling; hives; *superinfection; rash and other allergic reactions*

Chloramphenicol. See *Infection*

Chlorpheniramine maleate. See *Allergies*

Chlorpheniramine maleate, phenylpropanolamine hydro-chloride, isopropamide iodide $\boxed{\text{I}}$

Brand: Ornade (Smith Kline & French)

Capsule

Indications: upper respiratory congestion; inflammation of nose; allergy

Actions: reduces congestion and inflammation (antihistamine); lessens secretion of mucus; dries nasal passages

Possible side effects: anorexia; nausea; vomiting; diarrhea; constipation; drowsiness; lightheadedness; dry mouth, nose, and throat; blurred vision; nervousness; confusion; headache; insomnia; *urinary difficulties; muscle spasms; *photosensitivity; *irregular heart rhythm with palpitations; *bone marrow depression; rash and other allergic reactions*

Note: take 1/2–1 hour before food

Codeine phosphate, guaifenesin, pseudoephedrine hydro-chloride, triprolidine hydrochloride. See *Respiratory System*

Codeine sulfate, bromodiphenhydramine hydrochloride, diphenhydramine hydrochloride, ammonium chloride, potassium guaiacolsulfonate $\boxed{\text{C}}$ $\boxed{\text{D}}$ $\boxed{\text{F}}$ $\boxed{\text{I}}$

Brand: Ambenyl Expectorant (Marion)

Liquid

Indication: cough from cold and allergy

Actions: reduces congestion and inflammation (antihistamine); loosens phlegm; suppresses cough; relieves pain

Possible side effects: anorexia; nausea; vomiting; diarrhea; constipation; drowsiness; lightheadedness; dry mouth, nose, and throat; blurred vision; nervousness; confusion; headache; insomnia; *urinary difficulties; muscle spasms; *photosensitivity; *irregular heart rhythm with palpitations; *bone marrow depression; rash and other allergic reactions*

Colistin sulfate, neomycin sulfate, thonzonium bromide, hydrocortisone acetate

Brand: Coly-Mycin S Otic (Parke-Davis)

Liquid (topical)

Indication: infections of the external ear canal

Actions: treats infection; reduces inflammation

Possible side effects: allergic reactions with swelling and

redness

Dexamethasone. See *Musculo-Skeletal System*

Dexbrompheniramine maleate, pseudoephedrine sulfate

C   I

Brand: Drixoral (Schering)

Tablet

Indications: allergic skin reactions; congestion of sinus, ear, or respiratory system

Action: reduces congestion and inflammation (antihistamine)

Possible side effects: anorexia; nausea; vomiting; diarrhea; constipation; drowsiness; lightheadedness; dry mouth, nose, and throat; blurred vision; nervousness; confusion; headache; insomnia; muscle spasms; *irregular heart rhythm with palpitations; rash and other allergic reactions*

Note: pill must be swallowed whole

Dexchlorpheniramine maleate. See *Allergies*

Hydrocortisone. See *Musculo-Skeletal System*

Neomycin sulfate, hydrocortisone, acetic acid

Brand: Otic Neo-Cort-Dome (Dome)

Liquid (topical)

Indication: bacterial infections of external ear canal

Actions: treats bacterial infection; reduces inflammation

Possible side effects: allergic reactions with swelling and redness

Phenylpropanolamine hydrochloride, phenylephrine hydrochloride, phenyltoloxamine citrate, chlorpheniramine maleate F

Brand: Naldecon (Bristol)

Tablet, Liquid

Indications: cold symptoms; upper respiratory infection; allergy

Action: reduces congestion and inflammation (antihistamine)

Possible side effects: anorexia; nausea; vomiting; diarrhea; constipation; drowsiness; lightheadedness; dry mouth, nose, and throat; blurred vision; nervousness; headache; insomnia; *urinary difficulties; irregular heart rhythm with palpitations; rash and other allergic reactions*

Polymyxin B, neomycin, hydrocortisone

Brand: Cortisporin Otic (Burroughs Wellcome)

Liquid (topical)

Indication: bacterial infections of external ear canal

Actions: treats bacterial infection; reduces inflammation

Possible side effects: allergic reactions with swelling and redness

Promethazine hydrochloride, potassium guaiacolsulfonate

I

Brand: Phenergan Expectorant (Wyeth)

Liquid

Indication: cough from cold, allergy, and congestion

Actions: reduces congestion and inflammation (antihistamine); suppresses cough

Possible side effects: anorexia; nausea; vomiting; diarrhea; constipation; drowsiness; lightheadedness; dry mouth, nose, and throat; blurred vision; nervousness; confusion; headache; insomnia; *urinary difficulties; muscle spasms; photosensitivity; irregular heart rhythm with palpitations; bone marrow depression; rash and other allergic reactions*

Promethazine hydrochloride, potassium guaiacolsulfonate,

codeine phosphate ⃞D⃞ ⃞I⃞

Brand: Phenergan Expectorant with Codeine (Wyeth)

Liquid

Indication: cough and congestion from cold and allergy

Actions: reduces congestion and inflammation (antihistamine); suppresses cough; relieves pain

Possible side effects: anorexia; nausea; vomiting; diarrhea; constipation; drowsiness; lightheadedness; dry mouth, nose, and throat; blurred vision; nervousness; confusion; headache; insomnia; *urinary difficulties; muscle spasms; *photosensitivity; *irregular heart rhythm with palpitations; *bone marrow depression; rash and other allergic reactions*

Promethazine hydrochloride, potassium guaiacolsulfonate, phenylephrine hydrochloride ⃞F⃞ ⃞I⃞

Brand: Phenergan VC Expectorant (Wyeth)

Liquid

Indication: cough and congestion from cold and allergy

Actions: reduces congestion and inflammation (antihistamine); suppresses cough

Possible side effects: anorexia; nausea; vomiting; diarrhea; constipation; drowsiness; lightheadedness; dry mouth, nose, and throat; blurred vision; nervousness; confusion; headache; insomnia; *urinary difficulties; muscle spasms; *photosensitivity; *hepatitis; irregular heart rhythm with palpitations; *bone marrow depression; rash and other allergic reactions*

Promethazine hydrochloride, potassium guaiacolsulfonate, phenylephrine hydrochloride, codeine phosphate ⃞D⃞ ⃞F⃞ ⃞I⃞

Brand: Phenergan VC Expectorant with Codeine (Wyeth)

Liquid

Indication: cough and congestion from cold and allergy

Actions: reduces congestion and inflammation (antihistamine); suppresses cough; relieves pain

Possible side effects: anorexia; nausea; vomiting; diarrhea; constipation; drowsiness; lightheadedness; dry mouth, nose, and throat; blurred vision; nervousness; confusion; headache; insomnia; *urinary difficulties; muscle spasms; *photosensitivity; *irregular heart rhythm with palpitations; *bone marrow depression; rash and other allergic reactions*

Pseudoephedrine hydrochloride, triprolidine hydrochloride ⃞I⃞

Brand: Actifed (Burroughs Wellcome)

Tablet, Liquid

Indication: cough and congestion from cold and allergy

Action: reduces congestion and inflammation (antihistamine)

Possible side effects: anorexia; nausea; vomiting; diarrhea; constipation; drowsiness; lightheadedness; dry mouth, nose, and throat; blurred vision; nervousness; confusion; headache; insomnia; *urinary difficulties; muscle spasms; *photosensitivity; *irregular heart rhythm with palpitations; *bone marrow depression; rash and other allergic reactions*

Sulfamethoxazole. See *Infection*

NONPRESCRIPTION DRUGS

Alka-Seltzer Plus. See *Respiratory System*

Allerest. See *Allergies*

A.R.M. Allergy Relief Medicine. See *Allergies*

Bayer Children's Cold Tablets. See *Respiratory System*
Bayer Cough Syrup for Children. See *Respiratory System*
Cēpacol Mouthwash/Gargle (Merrell-National)
Liquid
Indications: dryness; throat irritation; odor
Actions: relieves dryness and throat irritation; reduces odor
Cēpacol Throat Lozenges (Merrell-National)
Lozenge
Indications: irritated mouth and throat; cough
Action: relieves cough and mouth and throat irritation
Cēpastat (Merrell-National)
Mouthwash, Lozenge
Indications: sore throat; mouth irritation; odor
Actions: relieves sore throat and mouth irritations; reduces odor
Chloraseptic. See *Mouth and Teeth*
Chloraseptic Children's Lozenges (Norwich-Eaton)
Lozenge
Indications: sore throat; mouth and gum irritation
Action: relieves pain and irritation
Chloraseptic DM Cough Control Lozenges (Norwich-Eaton)
Lozenge
Indications: sore throat; cough
Action: relieves pain and cough
Chlor-Trimeton. See *Respiratory System*
Chlor-Trimeton Allergy Syrup and Tablets. See *Allergies*
Comtrex. See *Respiratory System*
Congespirin. See *Respiratory System*
Coricidin. See *Respiratory System*
Coricidin Sinus Headache Tablets (Extra Strength) (Schering)
Tablet
Indications: headache; sinus congestion
Actions: relieves sinus pain; reduces congestion
Coryban-D. See *Respiratory System*
CoTylenol. See *Respiratory System*
Datril. See *Pain*
Dristan. See *Respiratory System*
Fedahist. See *Respiratory System*
Formula 44 Cough Control Discs (Vicks)
Tablet
Indications: sore throat; cough during cold, flu, and bronchitis
Actions: soothes throat; suppresses cough
Formula 44D Decongestant Cough Mixture. See *Respiratory System*
4-Way. See *Respiratory System*
Murine Ear Wax Removal System/Murine Ear Drops (Abbott)
Liquid
Indication: hardened ear wax
Actions: softens and loosens accumulated ear wax
Neo-Synephrine. See *Respiratory System*
Novahistine and Novahistine Sinus Tablets. See *Allergies*
Novahistine Cough Formula and Novahistine DMX. See *Respiratory System*
Nyquil Nighttime Colds Medicine. See *Respiratory System*
Primatene. See *Respiratory System*
Rhinosyn-DM, Rhinosyn-X. See *Respiratory System*
Rhinosyn Syrup, Rhinosyn-PD (Additive Free) (Comatic)
Liquid

Indication: nasal and sinus congestion
Action: relieves congestion
St. Joseph Cold Tablets for Children. See *Respiratory System*
St. Joseph Cough Syrup for Children. See *Respiratory System*
Sinarest Tablets. See *Allergies*
Sine-Aid Sinus Headache Tablets (McNeil)
Tablet
Indication: sinus headache and congestion
Actions: relieves pain; reduces congestion
Sine-Off. See *Allergies*
Sine-Off Once-A-Day Sinus Spray. See *Respiratory System*
Sinutab. See *Allergies*
Sinutab Long Lasting Decongestant Nasal Spray. See *Respiratory System*
Sinutab Tablets (Warner-Lambert)
Tablet
Indication: sinus headache and congestion
Action: reduces congestion and inflammation (antihistamine)
Sinutab-II Tablets (Warner-Lambert)
Tablet
Indications: headache; sinus congestion
Actions: relieves pain; reduces congestion
Sucrets (Beecham)
Lozenge
Indications: sore throat; oral irritation
Action: relieves sore throat and mouth irritation
Sucrets Cold Decongestant Formula (Beecham)
Lozenge
Indications: throat irritation; nasal congestion
Actions: relieves sore throat; reduces nasal congestion
Sucrets Cough Control Formula (Beecham)
Lozenge
Indications: throat irritation; cough
Actions: relieves throat irritation; suppresses cough
Symptom 2. See *Respiratory System*
Symptom 3. See *Allergies*
Triaminic. See *Respiratory System*
Triaminic Syrup. See *Allergies*
Triaminicin Tablets. See *Allergies*
Triaminicol Decongestant Cough Syrup. See *Respiratory System*
Vicks Cough Silencers Cough Drops (Vicks)
Lozenge
Indications: sore throat; cough
Actions: soothes throat; suppresses cough
Vicks Cough Syrup. See *Respiratory System*
Vicks Sinex Long-Acting Decongestant Nasal Spray. See *Allergies*

Eyes

Nonprescription eye drops can be helpful in reducing the redness caused by eye irritants, such as smoke and smog. However, these drops are not sufficient treatment for infections. If the eyes become swollen or purulent from an infection, a doctor should be consulted. Prescription eye medications (ointment or solution) have an anti-inflammatory agent, an antibiotic agent, or both. The anti-inflammatory agent reduces the swelling and redness, while the antibiotic agent attacks the disease-causing bacteria. Antibiotic drops tend to cause less blurriness and are therefore often preferred for use during the day, while antibiotic ointments are usually taken at night before sleep.

Using the correct method of applying eye drops or ointment will increase the medicine's effectiveness. Follow this procedure:

Drops

1. Ask someone else to assist if necessary.
2. Wash and dry hands thoroughly.
3. To prevent contamination, do not touch dropper to eye, face, or anything else.
4. Lie down on back on bed or couch.
5. Tilt head backward (for example, over side of bed).
6. With one hand pull down lower eyelid to form pouch.
7. With other hand hold dropper and approach eye from side (out of view), bringing dropper as close to eye as possible while still out of eye's view.
8. Drop into pouch the prescribed number of drops.
9. Close eyes (do not rub).
10. Squeeze bridge of nose gently (prevents eyedrops from draining).
11. Blot excess drops off face with tissue.
12. Repeat with other eye if so prescribed.

Ointment

Eye ointment is applied in the same manner except the prescribed amount is squeezed along the inside of the pouch.

Even if only one eye is infected, antibiotic drops or ointment are usually suggested for both eyes to treat an infection not yet apparent in the seemingly unaffected eye or to prevent the infection from spreading. Sometimes the infection does not respond to the prescribed antibiotic because the germ is resistant. If no improvement is apparent in the first 48 hours, the doctor should be informed.

Unlike eye irritation or infection, glaucoma may cause no apparent symptoms. This illness leads to pressure building up within the eye and can cause blindness if left untreated. Part of a routine physical examination should therefore include having the doctor measure eye pressure. If glaucoma (increased pressure) exists, daily eyedrops will be helpful. The drops must be taken regularly as prescribed, despite the apparent lack of any eye problem. Some medicines, such as certain antidepressants or cold medicines, can make glaucoma worse; drug labels and doctors should be consulted before taking a new drug.

PRESCRIPTION DRUGS

Acetazolamide. See *Cardiovascular System*
Chloramphenicol
Brand: Chloromycetin Ophthalmic (Parke-Davis)
Ointment
Indication: bacterial eye infections
Action: treats bacterial infections
Possible side effects: blurred vision; *rash and other allergic reactions*
Echothiophate

Brand: Phospholine Iodine (Ayerst)
Liquid (topical)
Indication: glaucoma
Action: reduces internal pressure of the eye
Possible side effects: blurred vision; *irritation of the eye;
   iris cysts*

Gentamicin sulfate
Brand: Garamycin Ophthalmic (Schering)
Liquid (topical), Ointment
Indications: bacterial eye infections; conjunctivitis; corneal
   ulcers
Action: treats bacterial infection
Possible side effects: blurred vision; irritation; burning or
   stinging; *rash and other allergic reactions*

Hydroxyamphetamine hydrobromide
Brand: Paredrine 1% (Smith Kline & French)
Liquid (topical)
Indication: need for pupil dilation (for eye examination)
Action: dilates pupils
Possible side effects: discomfort in bright light; blurred
   vision; *increased eye pressure*

Idoxuridine
Brand: Stoxil (Smith Kline & French)
Liquid (topical), Ointment
Indication: inflammation of the cornea from herpes
   simplex
Action: treats viral infections
Possible side effects: irritation; itching; pain; extreme
   sensitivity to light; *rash and other allergic reactions*

Neomycin sulfate, polymyxin B sulfate, zinc bacitracin
Brand: Neo-Polycin Ophthalmic (Dow)
Ointment
Indication: bacterial eye infections
Action: treats bacterial infection
Possible side effects: blurred vision; *rash and other allergic
   reactions*

Pilocarpine hydrochloride   ☐ I
Brand: Isopto-Carpine (Alcon)
Liquid (topical)
Indications: elevated eye pressure; glaucoma
Actions: constricts pupil; reduces internal pressure of the eye
Possible side effects: initial increase in eye pressure; blurred
   vision; itching of eyes and eyelids; *headache; tremors;
   palpitations; wheezing*

Polymyxin B, bacitracin
Brand: Polysporin Ointment Ophthalmic (Burroughs
   Wellcome)
Ointment
Indication: bacterial eye infections
Action: treats bacterial infection
Possible side effects: blurred vision; *superinfection; *rash
   and other allergic reactions*

Polymyxin B, bacitracin, neomycin, hydrocortisone
Brand: Cortisporin Ophthalmic (Burroughs Wellcome)
Ointment
Indications: bacterial eye infections; allergic conjunctivitis;
   corneal abrasions or burns
Actions: reduces inflammation; relieves itching; treats
   bacterial infection
Possible side effects: *rash and other allergic reactions*

Polymyxin B, neomycin, gramicidin

Brand: Neosporin Ophthalmic (Burroughs Wellcome)
Liquid (topical)

Indication: bacterial eye infections
Action: treats bacterial infection
Possible side effects: blurred vision; *rash and other allergic reactions*

Prednisolone acetate, sulfacetamide sodium
Brand: Metimyd (Schering)
Ointment, Liquid (topical)

Indication: infection and allergic inflammation of eye and eyelid
Actions: treats infection; reduces inflammation
Possible side effects: blurred vision; stinging; burning; *rash and other allergic reactions*

Prednisolone sodium phosphate
Brand: Metreton (Schering)
Liquid (topical).

Indication: allergy and inflammation of the eye
Action: reduces inflammation
Possible side effects: blurred vision; stinging; *cataract formation; secondary infections; glaucoma*

Prednisolone sodium phosphate, sulfacetamide sodium
Brand: Optimyd (Schering)
Liquid (topical)

Indications: infection and allergic inflammation of eye and eyelid
Actions: treats infection; reduces inflammation
Possible side effects: stinging; irritation; *rash and other allergic reactions*
See also listing for Prednisolone sodium phosphate

Silver nitrate
Generic manufacturer: Lilly
Liquid (topical)

Indication: prevention of eye infection in newborns
Action: prevents infection
Possible side effects: localized black staining

Sulfamethoxazole. See *Infection*
Sulfisoxazole diolamine
Brand: Gantrisin Ophthalmic (Roche)
Liquid (topical), Ointment

Indications: conjunctivitis; corneal ulcer; bacterial eye infections
Action: treats bacterial infection
Possible side effects: blurred vision; *superinfection; rash and other allergic reactions*

Timolol maleate
Brand: Timoptic (Merck Sharp & Dohme)
Liquid (topical)

Indication: glaucoma
Action: reduces internal pressure of the eye
Possible side effects: irritation; *rash and other allergic reactions*

Vidarabine
Brand: Vira-A (Parke-Davis)
Ointment

Indications: corneal conjunctivitis or inflammation due to herpes simplex virus
Action: treats viral infection
Possible side effects: blurred vision; irritation; sensitivity to light; *corneal inflammation*

NONPRESCRIPTION DRUGS

Clear Eyes (Abbott)
Liquid (topical)
Indication: eye irritation
Actions: moisturizes; soothes; reduces redness

Contique Cleaning and Soaking Solution (Alcon/bp)
Liquid (soaking solution)
Indication: hard contact lenses
Action: cleans hard contact lenses

Flexsol (Alcon/bp)
Liquid (soaking solution)
Indication: soft contact lenses
Actions: cleans and stores soft contact lenses

Lens-Mate (Alcon/bp)
Liquid (soaking solution; topical)
Indication: discomfort from hard contact lenses
Actions: cleans hard contact lenses; soothes eyes

Liquifilm Tears (Allergan)
Liquid (topical)
Indications: discomfort from hard contact lenses; dry eyes
Actions: lubricates and soothes eyes

Murine Eye Drops (Abbott)
Liquid (topical)
Indications: discomfort from contact lenses; eye irritation; eyestrain
Action: soothes eyes

Murine Plus Eye Drops (Abbott)
Liquid (topical)
Indication: eye irritation
Actions: soothes eyes; reduces redness

Preflex (Alcon/bp)
Liquid (cleaning solution)
Indication: soft contact lenses
Actions: cleans and disinfects soft contact lenses

Prefrin Liquifilm (Allergan)
Liquid (topical)
Indication: eye irritation
Actions: lubricates and soothes eyes; reduces redness

20/20 Eye Drops (S.S.S.)
Liquid (topical)
Indication: eye irritation
Action: reduces redness; soothes irritated eyes

Visine Eye Drops (Leeming)
Liquid (topical)
Indication: eye irritation
Actions: reduces redness; soothes irritated eyes

Gastrointestinal System

Many individuals become preoccupied with the normal day-to-day variations in the digestive system. Occasional nausea, gas, heartburn, diarrhea, or delayed bowel movements are normal. Drug treatment for these mild symptoms may lead to an overcompensation in the system and only perpetuate the digestive problem and the individual's concern.

Laxatives, for example, can be dangerous in some instances. They should not be taken during an acute gastrointestinal infection such as appendicitis. They can also cause diarrhea, dependence, and disturbances in the body chemistry. Laxatives work in different ways. Some stimulate the action of the gastrointestinal tract while others aid in the formation of bulk. Drugs that are stool softeners may take days to work.

On the other hand, certain symptoms are noteworthy and require consultation with a doctor. These symptoms include: persistent unrelieved pain, particularly if localized to a specific area; vomiting blood or coffee-ground appearing material (digested blood); pitch black stool (the color of tar, also digested blood); and bright red blood in the toilet bowl or on the tissue. The individual should not presume chronic hemorrhoids is the cause of bleeding until examined thoroughly by a doctor. Finally, any change in bowel habits lasting weeks and not just days should be evaluated.

PRESCRIPTION DRUGS

Apomorphine hydrochloride
Generic manufacturer: Lilly

Tablet

Indications: drug overdosage; poisoning by noncorrosive substances

Action: induces vomiting

Possible side effects: drowsiness; weakness; restlessness; tremors; *violent vomiting; rapid heartbeat; extremely low blood pressure*

Chlordiazepoxide hydrochloride, clidinium bromide D I
Brand: Librax (Roche)

Capsule

Indications: peptic ulcer; irritable bowel syndrome; inflammation of intestines

Actions: relieves anxiety; reduces gastric secretion and spasm

Possible side effects: nausea; constipation; drowsiness; dry mouth; blurred vision; *urinary difficulties; *blood and *liver disorders*

Cimetidine
Brand: Tagamet (Smith Kline & French)

Tablet, Injection

Indication: duodenal ulcer

Action: reduces gastric secretion

Possible side effects: diarrhea; dizziness; muscle aches; breast enlargement; slowed heartbeat; *blood disorders; rash and other allergic reactions*

Dicyclomine hydrochloride
Brand: Bentyl (Merrell-National)

Capsule, Tablet, Liquid, Injection

Indications: irritable or spastic colon; mucous colitis; acute enterocolitis; infant colic

Action: reduces gastric secretion and spasm

Possible side effects: nausea; vomiting; constipation; drowsiness; dry mouth; blurred vision; irritability; confusion; *urinary difficulties; *rapid heartbeat with palpitations; rash and other allergic reactions*

Diphenoxylate hydrochloride, atropine sulfate D I
Brand: Lomotil (Searle)

Tablet, Liquid

Indication: diarrhea

Action: relieves diarrhea

Possible side effects: anorexia; nausea; vomiting; dry mouth or nasal passages; flushed or red face; drowsiness; dizziness; headache; depression; *urinary difficulties; *irregular heartbeat; respiratory difficulty; numbness of hands and feet; fever; rash and other allergic reactions*

Common Gastrointestinal Problems

Symptoms	Possible Causes	Possible Treatments	Precautions
heartburn acid indigestion upper abdominal pain intolerance to spicy foods or coffee regurgitation	hiatus hernia duodenal ulcer gastritis anxiety	neutralize stomach acid with antacids reduce muscle spasm of stomach and intestines with antispasmodics avoid spicy, acidic foods and nicotine, coffee, and alcohol frequent small meals mild tranquilizers	antacids and antispasmodics may cause constipation mild tranquilizers may cause physical and psychological dependence chronicity and/or severity always indicate medical evaluation for serious underlying illness
intolerance of fatty foods pain under right ribs after eating bloating, burps, gas	gall bladder disease esophageal spasm	avoid fatty foods and dairy products reduce bloating with antigas medication surgical removal of inflamed or dysfunctional gallbladder	gallbladder stones may indicate high cholesterol levels underlying liver disease may be cause of symptoms medical evaluation advised
diarrhea	food allergy or "poisoning" virus infection nervous tension	maintain adequate fluid and salt intake avoid milk products during infectious bouts reduce intestinal contractions with antispasmodics, kaolin-pectin mixture	prolonged diarrhea causes dehydration and weakness diarrhea may be sign of appendicitis, ulcerative colitis, diverticulitis, or other serious illness medical evaluation advised
constipation	reduced ingestion of fiber limited physical activity nervousness or depression laxative dependence insufficient water intake unbalanced diet	increase intake of fiber and fruits increase intestinal bulk stool softeners laxatives increase water intake	change in bowel habits or stools is early sign of cancer of colon laxatives may be habit forming daily bowel movements are not necessary

Doxylamine succinate, pyridoxine hydrochloride [1]
Brand: Bendectin (Merrell-National)
Tablet
Indications: nausea and vomiting of pregnancy
Action: reduces nausea
Possible side effects: diarrhea; drowsiness; nervousness; headache
Warning: may cause birth defects
Erythromycin. See *Infection*
Hydrocortisone acetate, bismuth subgallate, bismuth resorcin, benzyl benzoate, Peruvian balsam, zinc oxide
Brand: Anusol-HC (Parke-Davis)
Cream, Suppository
Indications: hemorrhoids; anal itch
Action: reduces inflammation
Possible side effects: local irritation; dizziness; increased eye pressure

Ipecac
Generic manufacturer: Lilly
Liquid
Indications: drug overdosage; poisoning by noncorrosive
   substances
Action: induces vomiting
Possible side effects: stomach irritation; diarrhea; *severe
   vomiting with resulting palpitations*
Warning: seek advice of doctor, poison control center, or
   hospital emergency room before using

Kanamycin. See *Infection*

Mebendazole. See *Infection*

Meclizine hydrochloride [I]
Brand: Antivert (Roerig)
Tablet
Indications: nausea; vomiting; motion sickness; vertigo
Action: reduces nausea and dizziness
Possible side effects: drowsiness; dry mouth; blurred vision

Metronidazole. See *Urogenital System*

Opium (paregoric), pectin, kaolin [D] [I]
Brand: Parepectolin (Rorer)
Liquid
Indications: diarrhea; intestinal cramps
Action: relieves diarrhea
Possible side effects: nausea; vomiting; dizziness; drowsiness;
   lightheadedness; perspiring; *rash and other allergic reac-
   tions*

Paregoric [D] [I]
Generic manufacturers: Purepac, Rexall, Rorer
Liquid
Indication: diarrhea
Action: relieves diarrhea
Possible side effects: nausea; vomiting; dizziness; drowsi-
   ness; lightheadedness; perspiring; *rash and other allergic
   reactions*

**Phenobarbital, hyoscyamine sulfate, atropine sulfate,
hyoscine hydrobromide** [D] [I]
Brand: Donnatal (Robins)
Tablet, Capsule, Liquid
Indications: peptic ulcer; irritable bowel syndrome; intestinal inflammation; motion sickness
Actions: reduces gastric secretion and spasm; sedates
Possible side effects: nausea; vomiting; diarrhea; constipation; dry mouth; dry skin; lightheadedness; blurred
   vision; *urinary difficulties; impotence; *photosensitivity; *irregular heartbeat; hepatitis; *blood disorders;
   glaucoma; rash and other allergic reactions*

Piperazine. See *Infection*

Potassium chloride. See *Cardiovascular System*

Prochlorperazine [I]
Brand: Compazine (Smith Kline & French)
Tablet, Capsule, Injection, Suppository, Liquid
Indications: nausea; vomiting; anxiety; psychotic disorders
Actions: reduces nausea and vomiting; tranquilizes
Possible side effects: nausea; constipation; dry mouth;
   lightheadedness; drowsiness; restlessness; *photosensitivity; *urinary difficulties; impotence and retarded
   ejaculation; menstrual changes; breast enlargement;
   irregular heartbeat; tremors; *involuntary movements of
   face, jaw, tongue, and mouth; *bone marrow depression; *liver disorders; rash and other allergic reactions*

Prochlorperazine, isopropamide iodide   [I]
Brand: Combid (Smith Kline & French)
Capsule
Indications: peptic ulcer; irritable or spastic colon; mucous colitis; gastrointestinal disorders; diarrhea
Actions: reduces gastric secretions, spasm, and nausea; relieves anxiety
Possible side effects: nausea; constipation; dry mouth; lightheadedness; drowsiness; restlessness; *photosensitivity; *urinary difficulties; impotence and retarded ejaculation; menstrual changes; breast enlargement; irregular heartbeat; tremors; *involuntary movements of face, jaw, tongue, and mouth; *bone marrow depression; *liver disorders; rash and other allergic reactions*
See also listing for Prochlorperazine

Propantheline bromide
Brand: Pro-Banthine (Searle)
Tablet
Indications: peptic ulcer; irritable bowel syndrome
Action: reduces gastric secretion and spasm
Possible side effects: nausea; dry mouth; blurred vision; loss of sense of taste; drowsiness; nervousness; confusion; headache; dizziness; insomnia; *urinary difficulties; impotence; decreased perspiration; *irregular heartbeat; rash and other allergic reactions*

Pyrantel pamoate. See *Infection*

Simethicone, phenobarbital   [B] [D] [F] [I]
Brand: Phazyme-PB (Reed & Carnrick)
Tablet
Indication: gas pain
Action: releases gas; tranquilizes
Possible side effects: nausea; vomiting; diarrhea; constipation; *kidney disorders; blood pressure changes; rash and other allergic reactions*

Trimethobenzamide hydrochloride   [I]
Brand: Tigan (Beecham)
Capsule, Suppository, Injection
Indications: nausea; vomiting
Action: reduces nausea and vomiting
Possible side effects: diarrhea; drowsiness; dizziness; blurred vision; confusion; headache; *blood disorders; rash and other allergic reactions*

Trimethoprim, sulfamethoxazole. See *Urogenital System*
Vancomycin hydrochloride. See *Infection*

NONPRESCRIPTION DRUGS

Agoral (Parke-Davis)
Mineral Oil
Indication: constipation
Actions: relieves constipation; softens stool; lubricates

Alka-Seltzer Effervescent Antacid (Miles)
Tablet
Indications: acid indigestion; heartburn; upset stomach
Action: neutralizes excess stomach acid

Alka-Seltzer Effervescent Antacid & Analgesic (Miles)
Tablet
Indications: upset stomach; acid indigestion; heartburn; headache; aches and pains; fever
Actions: neutralizes excess stomach acid; reduces fever; relieves pain

Alka-2 (Miles)
Tablet
Indications: acid indigestion; upset stomach; heartburn
Action: neutralizes excess stomach acid
Allimin Filmcoated Tablets (Health Care)
Tablet
Indication: stomach and intestinal gas associated with intestinal spasm
Action: relaxes spasm
Aludrox (Wyeth)
Liquid, Tablet
Indications: heartburn; acid indigestion; hiatal hernia
Action: neutralizes excess stomach acid
Basaljel (Wyeth)
Liquid, Capsule
Indication: acid indigestion
Action: neutralizes excess stomach acid
Bisodol (Whitehall)
Tablet, Powder
Indications: heartburn; upset stomach; indigestion
Action: neutralizes excess stomach acid
Bonine (Pfipharmecs)
Tablet
Indication: motion sickness
Action: reduces motion sickness
Bu-lax, Bu-lax Plus (Ulmer)
Capsule
Indication: constipation
Actions: relieves constipation; softens stool
Camalox (Rorer)
Liquid, Tablet
Indication: increased stomach acidity
Action: neutralizes excess stomach acid
Carter's Little Pills (Carter)
Tablet
Indication: constipation
Action: relieves constipation by stimulating intestinal muscles
Charcocaps (Requa)
Capsule
Indications: diarrhea; gastrointestinal distress; gas
Actions: reduces irritants; absorbs intestinal gas
Correctol (Plough)
Tablet
Indication: constipation
Actions: relieves constipation; softens stool
Delcid (Merrell-National)
Liquid
Indication: increased stomach acidity
Action: neutralizes excess stomach acid
Derifil (Rystan)
Tablet, Powder
Indications: control of fecal and urinary odors associated with colostomy, ileostomy, or incontinence; body or breath odor
Action: deodorizes when taken by mouth or placed directly in the ostomy appliance
DeWitt's Antacid Powder (DeWitt)
Powder
Indications: acid indigestion; sour stomach; heartburn
Action: neutralizes excess stomach acid
Dicarbosil Antacid Tablets (Norcliff Thayer)

Tablet
Indication: increased stomach acidity
Action: neutralizes stomach acid

Di-Gel (Plough)
Tablet, Liquid
Indications: heartburn; indigestion; upset stomach; gas
Action: neutralizes excess stomach acid

Digestive Enzymes-PXP (Nion)
Tablet
Indication: digestive difficulties
Action: improves digestion

Dimenhydrinate Tablets (Lederle)
Tablet
Indication: motion sickness
Action: reduces motion sickness

Dorbane (Riker)
Tablet
Indication: constipation
Action: relieves constipation by stimulation of intestinal muscles

Dorbantyl Capsules, Dorbantyl Forte Capsules (Riker)
Capsule
Indication: constipation
Actions: relieves constipation by stimulation of intestinal muscles; softens stool

Dramamine, Dramamine Junior (Searle)
Tablet, Liquid
Indication: motion sickness
Action: reduces motion sickness

Dulcolax (Boehringer Ingelheim)
Tablet, Suppository
Indication: constipation
Action: relieves constipation by stimulating intestinal muscles

Emetrol (Rorer)
Liquid
Indications: nausea; vomiting
Action: reduces nausea and vomiting

Ex-Lax (Ex-Lax Pharm.)
Tablet, chocolate-flavored and unflavored
Indication: constipation
Action: relieves constipation

Gaviscon Liquid Antacid, Gaviscon Antacid Tablets, Gaviscon-2 Antacid Tablets (Marion)
Liquid, Tablet
Indications: heartburn; sour stomach; acid indigestion
Action: neutralizes excess stomach acid

Gelusil, Gelusil-II, Gelusil-M (Parke-Davis)
Liquid, Tablet
Indications: heartburn; sour stomach; acid indigestion; gas
Action: neutralizes excess stomach acid

Haley's M-O (Winthrop)
Liquid, regular and flavored
Indication: constipation
Actions: relieves constipation; lubricates

HTO Stainless Manzan Hemorrhoidal Tissue Ointment (DeWitt)
Ointment
Indication: hemorrhoids
Actions: lubricates; reduces swelling, inflammation, itching, and pain

Kaopectate, Kaopectate Concentrate (Upjohn)
Liquid
Indication: diarrhea
Action: reduces diarrhea
Kondremul (Fisons)
Liquid
Indication: constipation
Actions: relieves constipation; softens stool
Kudrox (Kremers-Urban)
Liquid, Tablet
Indications: heartburn; acid indigestion
Action: neutralizes excess stomach acid
Maalox Antacid, Maalox Plus Antacid-Antiflatulent, Maalox Therapeutic Concentrate (Rorer)
Tablet, Liquid
Indications: acid indigestion; gas
Action: neutralizes excess stomach acid
Metamucil, Instant Mix Metamucil, Orange Flavor Metamucil (Searle)
Powder
Indication: constipation
Actions: relieves constipation; acts as a bulk stimulant
Modane (Warren-Teed)
Tablet, Liquid
Indication: constipation
Action: relieves constipation
Modane Bulk (Warren-Teed)
Powder
Indication: constipation
Actions: relieves constipation; acts as a bulk laxative; softens stool
Modane Soft (Warren-Teed)
Capsule
Indication: constipation
Actions: relieves constipation; softens stool
Mylanta, Mylanta II (Stuart)
Liquid, Tablet
Indications: acid indigestion; gas
Action: neutralizes excess stomach acid
Neoloid (Lederle)
Liquid
Indication: constipation
Actions: relieves constipation; lubricates
Nupercainal (CIBA)
Ointment, Suppository, Cream
Indications: hemorrhoids; sunburn; insect bites; cuts; scratches; minor burns
Actions: lubricates; reduces swelling, inflammation, itching, and pain
Pancrelipase (Nion)
Tablet
Indication: digestive difficulty
Action: improves digestion
Pazo Hemorrhoid Ointment/Suppositories (Whitehall)
Ointment, Suppository
Indication: hemorrhoids
Actions: lubricates; reduces swelling, inflammation, itching, and pain
Pepto-Bismol (Norwich-Eaton)
Liquid, Tablet

Indications: upset stomach; indigestion; nausea; diarrhea
Actions: relieves nausea, gas pains, and cramps; reduces diarrhea

Peri-Colace (Mead Johnson)
Capsule
Indication: constipation
Actions: relieves constipation; softens stool

Phazyme, Phazyme-95 (Reed & Carnrick)
Tablet
Indication: intestinal gas pain
Action: releases intestinal gas

Phillips' Milk of Magnesia (Glenbrook)
Liquid
Indications: constipation; increased stomach acid
Actions: relieves constipation; neutralizes excess stomach acid

Preparation H Hemorrhoidal Ointment and Suppositories (Whitehall)
Ointment, Suppository
Indication: hemorrhoids
Actions: lubricates; reduces swelling, inflammation, itching, and pain

Rectal Medicone Suppositories (Medicone)
Suppository
Indication: hemorrhoids
Actions: lubricates; reduces swelling, inflammation, itching, and pain

Rectal Medicone Unguent (Medicone)
Ointment with applicator
Indication: hemorrhoids
Actions: lubricates; reduces swelling, inflammation, itching, and pain

Riopan (Ayerst)
Liquid, Tablet
Indications: heartburn; sour stomach; acid indigestion; increased stomach acid
Action: neutralizes excess stomach acid

Rolaids Antacid Tablets (Warner-Lambert)
Tablet
Indications: acid indigestion; heartburn; sour stomach
Action: neutralizes excess stomach acid

Syllact (Wallace)
Powder
Indication: constipation
Action: relieves constipation; acts as a bulk stimulant

Tums (Norcliff Thayer)
Tablet
Indications: acid indigestion; heartburn; sour stomach
Action: neutralizes excess stomach acid

Hormones

Hormones are secreted by different endocrine glands throughout the body to regulate metabolism, growth, reproduction, and other important functions. Drugs can replace these hormones when they are deficient (such as insulin for diabetes and thyroid for hypothyroidism) or they can block the functioning of these hormones (such as oral contraceptives for birth control). The endocrine system is held in delicate balance; any slight increase or decrease in the amount of hormone can affect the entire body. For this reason, great care must be taken in finding the proper drug dosage and under no circumstances should these drugs be taken casually without well-documented indications.

Diabetes
PRESCRIPTION DRUGS

Acetohexamide [1]
Brand: Dymelor (Lilly)
Tablet
Indication: Diabetes
Action: reduces blood sugar level by stimulating insulin secretion
Possible side effects: nausea; diarrhea; heartburn; headache; ringing in ears; *liver disorders with jaundice; *bone marrow depression; too low blood sugar with weakness and lightheadedness; rash and other allergic reactions*

Chlorpropamide [1]
Brand: Diabinese (Pfizer)
Tablet
Indication: diabetes
Action: reduces blood sugar level by stimulating insulin secretion
Possible side effects: anorexia; nausea; vomiting; diarrhea; too low blood sugar with weakness, lightheadedness, and headache; *liver disorders with jaundice; *bone marrow depression; rash and other allergic reactions*

Diazoxide
Brand: Proglycem (Schering)
Capsule, Liquid
Indication: low blood sugar due to high insulin
Action: increases blood sugar level
Possible side effects: anorexia; nausea; vomiting; diarrhea; flushing; excessive growth of facial and body hair; anxiety; dizziness; insomnia; *rapid heartbeat with palpitations; cataracts; rash and other allergic reactions*

Insulin NPH [1]
Brands: Isophane Insulin (Squibb), NPH Iletin (Lilly)
Injection
Indication: diabetes
Action: reduces blood sugar level by stimulating body to utilize sugar
Possible side effects: nausea; diarrhea; abdominal cramps; too low blood sugar with dizziness, drowsiness, shortness of breath, loss of consciousness; rash and other allergic reactions*

Potassium chloride. See Cardiovascular System
Protamine zinc insulin [1]
Brands: Protamine, Zinc & Iletin; Iletin Lente (Lilly)
Injection
Indication: diabetes
Action: reduces blood sugar level by stimulating body to use sugar
Possible side effects: nausea; diarrhea; abdominal cramps; too low blood sugar with dizziness, drowsiness, shortness of breath, loss of consciousness; rash and other allergic reactions*

Tolazamide [1]
Brand: Tolinase (Upjohn)

Tablet

Indication: adult-onset diabetes

Action: reduces blood sugar level by stimulating insulin secretion

Possible side effects: nausea; vomiting; weakness; fatigue; dizziness; vertigo; headache; **liver disorders with jaundice; *bone marrow depression; rash and other allergic reactions*

Warning: increased chance of heart problems

Tolbutamide $\boxed{1}$

Brand: Orinase (Upjohn)

Tablet

Indication: adult-onset diabetes

Action: reduces blood sugar level by stimulating insulin secretion

Possible side effects: nausea; diarrhea; heartburn; headache; **photosensitivity; *bone marrow depression; *liver disorders with jaundice; rash and other allergic reactions*

Sex Hormones

PRESCRIPTION DRUGS

Chlorotrianisene

Brand: TACE (Merrell-National)

Capsule

Indications: postpartum breast engorgement; cancer of prostate gland; menopausal disturbances

Action: helps prevent postpartum breast engorgement and menopausal disturbances; decreases prostate cancer by increasing estrogen level

Possible side effects: nausea; vomiting; fluid retention; weight gain or loss; nervousness; loss of hair or abnormal hair growth; headache; breast tenderness and enlargement; depression; change in potency or libido; *jaundice; rash and other allergic reactions*

Warning: possible **carcinogen*

Conjugated estrogen

Brand: Premarin Oral (Ayerst)

Tablet

Indications: menopausal disturbances; ovarian failure; postpartum breast engorgement; prostate and breast cancer; thinning and inflammation of vagina

Actions: regulates menstrual cycle; increases hormone level

Possible side effects: nausea; vomiting; bloating; weight gain or loss; fluid retention and edema; dizziness; mood changes; change or resumption of menstrual flow; breast enlargement or tenderness; **photosensitivity; skin discoloration; change in corneal curvature and intolerance to contact lenses; *liver disorders or gall bladder disease; increased risk of strokes*

Warning: possible **carcinogen* with prolonged usage; should not be used during pregnancy; potential risk of birth defects

Danazol

Brand: Danocrine (Winthrop)

Capsule

Indications: endometriosis; fibrocystic breast disease

Action: suppresses certain hormone secretions of pituitary gland

Possible side effects: nausea; vomiting; constipation; dizziness; headache; fatigue; sleep disorders; nervousness;

flushing; increased perspiring; vaginal itching; oiliness of skin or hair; acne; abnormal hair growth; weight gain; fluid retention; vision disturbances; *rash and other allergic reactions*

Diethylstilbestrol

Generic manufacturer: Lilly

Tablet, Vaginal suppository

Indications: menopausal disturbances; female hormone deficiency; breast and prostate cancer

Action: increases estrogen level

Possible side effects: nausea; vomiting; intestinal cramps; headache; dizziness; menstrual changes; breast tenderness and enlargement; loss of hair or abnormal hair growth; mood changes; fluid retention; weight gain or loss; discoloration and inflammation of the skin; increased risk of vaginal infections; **liver disorders and gall bladder disease with jaundice; increased risk of stroke*

Warning: possible *carcinogen with prolonged usage; should not be used during pregnancy; potential risk of birth defects

Ethinyl estradiol

Brand: Estinyl (Schering)

Tablet

Indications: menopausal disturbances; female hormone deficiency; breast and prostate cancer

Action: increases estrogen level

Possible side effects: nausea; vomiting; intestinal cramps; headache; dizziness; menstrual changes; breast tenderness and enlargement; loss of hair or abnormal hair growth; mood changes; fluid retention; weight gain or loss; discoloration and inflammation of the skin; increased risk of vaginal infections; **liver disorders and gall bladder disease with jaundice; increased risk of stroke*

Ethynodiol diacetate, ethinyl estradiol

Brand: Demulen (Searle)

Tablet

Indication: decrease chance of pregnancy

Action: prevents ovulation

Possible side effects: nausea; vomiting; headache; mood changes; menstrual changes and bleeding between cycles; temporary infertility after discontinuation; fluid retention; weight gain or loss; skin discoloration; changes in hair growth; breast tenderness, enlargement, or secretion; change in corneal curvature and intolerance to contact lenses; changes in cervical cells; *increased risk of phlebitis, high blood pressure, and stroke; *liver disorders and gall bladder disease with jaundice; increased risk of fetal abnormalities, including masculinization of females; rash and other allergic reactions*

See also listing for Ethinyl estradiol

Warning: possible *carcinogen with prolonged usage; should not be used during pregnancy; potential risk of birth defects

Ethynodiol diacetate, mestranol

Brand: Ovulen-21 (Searle)

Tablet

Indication: decrease chance of pregnancy

Action: prevents ovulation

Possible side effects: nausea; vomiting; breast tenderness, enlargement, or secretion; headache; mood changes; menstrual changes and bleeding between cycles; temporary infertility after discontinuation; fluid retention; weight gain or loss; skin discoloration; changes in hair growth; change in corneal curvature and intolerance to contact lenses; changes in cervical cells; *increased risk of phlebitis, high blood pressure, and stroke; *liver disorders and gall bladder disease with jaundice; increased risk of fetal abnormalities, including masculinization of females; rash and other allergic reactions*

Warning: possible *carcinogen with prolonged usage; should not be used during pregnancy; potential risk of birth defects

Medroxyprogesterone acetate
Brands: Provera, Depo-Provera (Upjohn)
Tablet
Indications: menstrual disorders; abnormal uterine bleeding; decrease chance of pregnancy
Action: prevents ovulation
Possible side effects: nausea; vomiting; headache; mood changes; menstrual changes and bleeding between cycles; temporary infertility after discontinuation; fluid retention; weight gain or loss; skin discoloration; changes in hair growth; breast tenderness, enlargement, or secretion; change in corneal curvature and intolerance to contact lenses; changes in cervical cells; *increased risk of phlebitis, high blood pressure, and stroke; *liver disorders and gall bladder disease with jaundice; increased risk of fetal abnormalities, including masculinization of females; rash and other allergic reactions*

Birth Control Methods

TYPE	HOW OBTAINED	FAILURE RATE PER YEAR	
		Method Failure	User Failure
oral contraceptive pill	prescription	less than 3%	3%
intrauterine device (IUD)	prescription	2—4%	none
diaphragm	prescription	2—4%	10—15%
condom	over the counter	2—4%	6—13%
contraceptive foam	over the counter	2—4%	13—16%
fertility awareness (rhythm)	education temperature chart	5—10%	9—28%
sterilization male female	surgical surgical	less than 1% less than 1%	none none

Warning: possible *carcinogen with prolonged usage; should not be used during pregnancy; potential risk of birth defects

Methyltestosterone

Brands: Oreton Methyl (Schering), Metandren (CIBA)

Tablet

Indications: androgen deficiency; male sexual underdevelopment; postpartum breast pain; breast cancer

Actions: increases androgen level; fights hormone-dependent breast tumor

Possible side effects: nausea; abnormal hair growth or baldness; sexual overstimulation; decrease in sperm production; male breast enlargement; masculinization of females; *liver disorders with jaundice; rash and other allergic reactions*

Norethindrone acetate

Brand: Norlutate (Parke-Davis)

Tablet

Indications: menstrual pain and irregularities; decrease chance of pregnancy; endometriosis

Actions: relieves painful periods; prevents ovulation

Possible side effects: nausea; vomiting; headache; mood changes; menstrual changes and bleeding between cycles; temporary infertility after discontinuation; fluid retention; weight gain or loss; skin discoloration; changes in hair growth; breast tenderness, enlargement, or secretion; change in corneal curvature and intolerance to contact lenses; changes in cervical cells; *increased risk of phlebitis, high blood pressure, and stroke; *liver disorders and gall bladder disease with jaundice; increased risk of fetal abnormalities, including masculinization of females; rash and other allergic reactions*

Warning: possible *carcinogen with prolonged usage; should not be used during pregnancy; potential risk of birth defects

Norethindrone acetate, ethinyl estradiol

Brand: Norlestrin 1/50-21 (Parke-Davis)

Tablet

Indication: decrease chance of pregnancy

Action: prevents ovulation

Possible side effects: nausea; vomiting; headache; mood changes; menstrual changes and bleeding between cycles; temporary infertility after discontinuation; fluid retention; weight gain or loss; skin discoloration; changes in hair growth; breast tenderness, enlargement, or secretion; change in corneal curvature and intolerance to contact lenses; changes in cervical cells; *increased risk of phlebitis, high blood pressure, and stroke; *liver disorders and gall bladder disease with jaundice; increased risk of fetal abnormalities, including masculinization of females; rash and other allergic reactions*
See also listings for Norethindrone acetate and Ethinyl estradiol

Warning: possible *carcinogen with prolonged usage; should not be used during pregnancy; potential risk of birth defects

Norethindrone, mestranol

Brands: Norinyl 1+50 21-Day (Syntex), Ortho-Novum 1/50-21, Ortho-Novum 1/80-21, Ortho-Novum 1/50-28 (Ortho)

Tablet

Indication: decrease chance of pregnancy

Action: prevents ovulation

Possible side effects: nausea; vomiting; headache; mood changes; menstrual changes and bleeding between cycles; temporary infertility after discontinuation; fluid retention; weight gain or loss; skin discoloration; changes in hair growth; breast tenderness, enlargement, or secretion; change in corneal curvature and intolerance to contact lenses; changes in cervical cells; *increased risk of phlebitis, high blood pressure, and stroke; *liver disorders and gall bladder disease with jaundice; increased risk of fetal abnormalities, including masculinization of females; rash and other allergic reactions*

Warning: possible *carcinogen with prolonged usage; should not be used during pregnancy; potential risk of birth defects

Norgestrel, ethinyl estradiol

Brands: Lo/Ovral, Ovral, Ovral-28 (Wyeth)

Tablet

Indication: decrease chance of pregnancy

Action: prevents ovulation

Possible side effects: nausea; vomiting; headache; mood changes; menstrual changes and bleeding between cycles; temporary infertility after discontinuation; fluid retention; weight gain or loss; skin discoloration; changes in hair growth; breast tenderness, enlargement, or secretion; change in corneal curvature and intolerance to contact lenses; changes in cervical cells; *increased risk of phlebitis, high blood pressure, and stroke; *liver disorders and gall bladder disease with jaundice; increased risk of fetal abnormalities, including masculinization of females; rash and other allergic reactions*
See also listing for Ethinyl estradiol

Warning: possible *carcinogen with prolonged usage; should not be used during pregnancy; potential risk of birth defects

Thyroid

PRESCRIPTION DRUGS

Dexamethasone. See Musculo-Skeletal System

Liothyronine sodium

Brand: Cytomel (Smith Kline & French)

Tablet

Indications: thyroid hormone deficiency; goiter; thyroid cancer

Action: replaces thyroid hormone

Possible side effects: headache; weight loss; tremors; insomnia; poor tolerance of heat; menstrual changes; *irregular heartbeat or angina pectoris with palpitations; rash and other allergic reactions*

Methimazole

Brand: Tapazole (Lilly)

Tablet

Indication: hyperthyroidism

Action: inhibits synthesis of thyroid hormones

Possible side effects: nausea; vomiting; dizziness; headache; loss of taste; muscle and joint pain; loss of hair; *susceptibility to infection; rash and other allergic reactions*

Propylthiouracil

Generic manufacturers: Lilly, American Pharmaceutical, Purepac
Tablet
Indication: hyperthyroidism
Action: suppresses thyroid function
Possible side effects: nausea; vomiting; headache; drowsiness; vertigo; loss of taste; muscle and joint pain; loss of hair; nerve inflammation and pain; fluid retention; *bone marrow depression; *liver disorders with jaundice; rash and other allergic reactions

Sodium levothyroxine
Brands: Levothroid (Armour), Synthroid (Flint)
Tablet, Injection
Indication: reduced or absent thyroid function
Action: replaces thyroid hormone
Possible side effects: headache; weight loss; tremors; insomnia; poor tolerance of heat; menstrual changes; *irregular heartbeat or angina pectoris with palpitations; rash and other allergic reactions*

Thyroglobulin
Brand: Proloid (Parke-Davis)
Tablet
Indication: thyroid hormone deficiency
Action: replaces thyroid hormone
Possible side effects: headache; weight loss; tremors; insomnia; poor tolerance of heat; menstrual changes; *irregular heartbeat or angina pectoris with palpitations; rash and other allergic reactions*

Thyroid
Brands: Armour Thyroid (Armour), Thyroid Strong (Marion), S-P-T (Fleet)
Tablet, Capsule
Indication: thyroid hormone deficiency
Action: replaces thyroid hormone
Possible side effects: headache; weight loss; tremors; insomnia; poor tolerance of heat; menstrual changes; *irregular heartbeat or angina pectoris with palpitations; rash and other allergic reactions*

Adrenal Hormones

PRESCRIPTION DRUGS

Fludrocortisone acetate
Brand: Florinef Acetate (Squibb)
Tablet
Indication: Addison's disease
Action: replaces adrenal hormones
Possible side effects: fluid retention; abnormal hair growth; menstrual changes; *decreased potassium levels with muscle weakness, high blood pressure, and heart failure; cataracts; rash and other allergic reactions*

Oxymetholone
Brands: Adroyd (Parke-Davis), Anadrol-50 (Syntex)
Tablet
Indication: anemia
Action: stimulates production of red blood cells
Possible side effects: nausea; abnormal hair growth or baldness; sexual overstimulation; decrease in sperm production; male breast enlargement; masculinization of females; *liver disorders with jaundice; rash and other allergic reactions*

Infection

"Germs" are tiny living organisms, such as viruses and bacteria. Many of these microorganisms *normally* can be found on the skin, in the mouth, in the intestinal system, even in the air we breathe. Only rarely do they cause an infection. The goal of drug treatment is therefore not to eliminate all microorganisms, which in fact play an important role in many of the body's functions, such as digestion. Instead, the goal of drug treatment for an infection is to *reduce* the number of a particularly virulent or powerful microorganism ("bug") so that the body's normal defensive processes can work effectively.

When taking these anti-infection (antibiotic) drugs, several general principles should be kept in mind. First, not all antibiotics work for all microorganisms. On the contrary, an antibiotic must be selected that specifically interferes with the growth of or kills the particular infective agent. A medicine that worked for one infection may not work for the next even if the infection is in the same area. Second, during the course of treatment the infective microorganisms may change their form and become resistant to the prescribed antibiotic. Another antibiotic may then become necessary. Third, an infection may still be present even *after* the symptoms have gone. To prevent a potentially dangerous smoldering infection, take the antibiotic for the prescribed number of days even though relief has occurred. Fourth, sometimes the infection—such as a common cold—is caused by a virus and no antibiotics are known that can reduce this particular infective agent. Taking an ineffective antibiotic can be hazardous because the chance of producing powerful and resistant microorganisms is increased. Therefore, antibiotics are not advised for self-limited illnesses for which no known anti-infective drugs are available. Fifth, infections often occur when the body is especially vulnerable or poorly defended. For example, the skin becomes infected in the area of a cut or the teeth become infected because of a cavity. When infections are recurrent, repeated use of antibiotics is not sufficient treatment. The underlying cause for the reduced resistance should be investigated.

PRESCRIPTION DRUGS

Amantadine. See *Nervous System*

Amoxicillin
Generic manufacturers: Premo, Comer
Brands: Amoxil (Beecham), Larotid (Roche), Polymox (Bristol), Wymox (Wyeth)
Capsule, Liquid
Indication: bacterial infections
Action: treats bacterial infections
Possible side effects: nausea; vomiting; diarrhea; *black tongue*; *blood disorders*; *rash and other allergic reactions*
Note: refrigerate liquid

Amphotericin B
Brand: Fungizone (Squibb)
Cream, Ointment, Lotion
Indications: topical fungal infections; ringworm
Action: treats fungal infections
Possible side effects: dryness; irritation; itching; burning

of the skin

Ampicillin
Generic manufacturers: Rexall, Purepac, Comer
Brands: Amcill (Parke-Davis), Omnipen (Wyeth), Polycillin (Bristol), Principen (Squibb)
Capsule, Powder, Liquid, Injection
Indication: bacterial infections
Action: treats bacterial infection
Possible side effects: nausea; vomiting; diarrhea; *blood disorders; rash and other allergic reactions*
Note: refrigerate liquid

Arsenic derivative
Brand: Carbarsone (Lilly)
Capsule
Indication: intestinal amebic infection
Action: treats amebic infection
Possible side effects: nausea; vomiting; diarrhea; abdominal cramps; *rash and other allergic reactions*

Carbenicillin
Brand: Geocillin (Roerig)
Tablet
Indication: infections, particularly of prostate and urinary tract
Action: treats bacterial infections
Possible side effects: nausea; vomiting; diarrhea; abdominal cramps; dry mouth; *blood disorders; rash and other allergic reactions*

Cephalexin
Brand: Keflex (Lilly)
Tablet, Capsule, Liquid
Indication: bacterial infections
Action: treats bacterial infections
Possible side effects: nausea; vomiting; diarrhea; *blood disorders; rash and other allergic reactions*
Note: refrigerate liquid

Chloramphenicol [1]
Brands: Amphicol (McKesson), Antibiopto (Softcon), Chloromycetin (Parke-Davis), Chloroptic (Allergan), Econochlor (Alcon), Mychel (Rachelle), Ophthochlor (Parke-Davis)
Capsule, Liquid, Cream
Indication: bacterial infections
Action: treats bacterial infections
Possible side effects: nausea; vomiting; diarrhea; headache; *black tongue; confusion; tingling in hands and feet; *superinfections; *bone marrow depression; rash and other allergic reactions*
Warning: should not be taken during pregnancy

Chloroquine phosphate
Brand: Aralen (Winthrop)
Tablet
Indication: parasitic infections, especially malaria
Action: treats parasitic infections
Possible side effects: anorexia; nausea; vomiting; diarrhea; abdominal cramps; headache; emotional disturbances; vision disturbances; *convulsions; deafness; *blood disorders; rash and other allergic reactions*

Clindamycin
Brand: Cleocin hydrochloride (Upjohn)
Capsule, Liquid
Indication: bacterial infections

Action: treats bacterial infections

Possible side effects: nausea; vomiting; diarrhea; abdominal pain; **liver and *blood disorders; rash and other allergic reactions*

Clotrimazole. See *Urogenital System*

Clotrimazole. See *Skin, Hair, and Scalp*

Colistin sulfate, neomycin sulfate, thonzonium bromide, hydrocortisone acetate. See *Ear, Nose, and Throat*

Cycloserine

Brand: Seromycin (Lilly)

Capsule

Indications: tuberculosis; resistant urinary infections

Action: treats bacterial infections

Possible side effects: nervous system symptoms, such as headache, drowsiness, convulsion, confusion, and emotional changes; rash and other allergic reactions

Diaminodiphenylsulfone (DDS)

Brand: Dapsone (Jacobus)

Tablet

Indication: leprosy

Action: treats leprosy infections

Possible side effects: nausea; vomiting; abdominal pain; ringing in ears; dizziness; headache; emotional disturbances; blurred vision; *photosensitivity; muscle weakness; **liver or *kidney disorders; *bone marrow depression; rash and other allergic reactions*

Dicloxacillin sodium

Brands: Dynapen (Bristol), Pathocil (Wyeth), Veracillin (Ayerst)

Capsule, Liquid

Indication: bacterial infections

Action: treats bacterial infections

Possible side effects: nausea; vomiting; abdominal discomfort; diarrhea; *rash and other allergic reactions*

Diiodohydroxyquin, hydrocortisone

Brand: Vytone Cream (Dermik)

Cream

Indications: skin rash and infection

Action: treats topical fungal and bacterial infections

Possible side effects: dry skin; rash with itching or burning; skin discoloration; *secondary infection*

Doxycycline   [I]

Brand: Vibramycin (Pfizer)

Capsule, Liquid

Indication: bacterial infections

Action: treats bacterial infections

Possible side effects: anorexia; diarrhea; vomiting; tongue inflammation; *photosensitivity; *superinfection; **liver, *blood, and *kidney disorders; rash and other allergic reactions*

Erythromycin   [I]

Brands: E-Mycin (Upjohn), Ilosone (Dista), Pediamycin (Ross) E.E.S., Erythrocin (Abbott)

Tablet, Capsule, Liquid, Granule

Indication: bacterial infections

Action: treats bacterial infections

Possible side effects: nausea; vomiting; diarrhea; abdominal pain; **superinfection: *liver disorders; rash and other allergic reactions*

Ethambutol hydrochloride

Brand: Myambutol (Lederle)

Tablet
Indication: tuberculosis
Action: treats bacterial infection
Possible side effects: anorexia; nausea; vomiting; abdominal pain; headache; dizziness; confusion; hallucinations; tingling of hands and feet; joint pain; aggravation of gout; *vision disturbances; *liver disorders; rash and other allergic reactions*

Gentamicin sulfate
Brand: Garamycin (Schering)
Cream, Ointment
Indication: bacterial skin infections
Action: treats topical bacterial infection
Possible side effects: irritation; *photosensitivity; *superinfection*

Griseofulvin [1]
Brands: Fulvicin (Schering), Grifulvin V (Ortho), Grisactin (Ayerst), Gris-PEG (Dorsey)
Tablet, Capsule, Liquid
Indication: ringworm infections
Action: treats fungal infections
Possible side effects: nausea; vomiting; diarrhea; headache; dizziness; confusion; insomnia; *photosensitivity; *superinfection; rash and other allergic reactions*

Idoxuridine. See *Eyes*

Isoniazid [1]
Brands: INH (CIBA), Nydrazid (Squibb)
Tablet, Capsule
Indication: tuberculosis
Action: treats tubercular infection
Possible side effects: nausea; vomiting; indigestion; tingling in hands and feet; muscle and joint pain; breast enlargement; vision disturbances; emotional disturbances; confusion; *convulsions; *liver disorders; *bone marrow depression; rash and other allergic reactions*
Warning: possible *carcinogen

Kanamycin
Brand: Kantrex (Bristol)
Capsule
Indication: bacterial infections
Action: treats bacterial infections
Possible side effects: nausea; vomiting; diarrhea; dizziness; ringing in ears; *ear and *kidney disorders; rash and other allergic reactions*

Lincomycin hydrochloride
Brand: Lincocin (Upjohn)
Capsule, Injection, Liquid
Indication: serious bacterial infections
Action: treats serious bacterial infections
Possible side effects: nausea; vomiting; diarrhea; abdominal cramps; tongue inflammation; skin discoloration; dizziness; ringing in ears; *liver and *blood disorders; rash and other allergic reactions*

Mebendazole
Brand: Vermox (Janssen)
Tablet
Indications: whipworm; pinworm; roundworm; hookworm
Action: treats worm infestation
Possible side effects: abdominal pain; diarrhea

Methenamine, phenyl salicylate, gelsemium, methylene blue, benzoic acid, atropine sulfate, hyoscyamine. See *Urogenital System*

Methenamine, phenyl salicylate, methylene blue, benzoic acid, atropine sulfate, hyoscyamine. See *Urogenital System*

Methenamine, sodium acid phosphate. See *Urogenital System*

Metronidazole. See *Urogenital System*

Miconazole nitrate. See *Urogenital System*

Minocycline hydrochloride   ☐ I

Brand: Minocin (Lederle)
Capsule, Liquid, Injection
Indication: bacterial infections
Action: treats bacterial infections
Possible side effects: anorexia; nausea; vomiting; diarrhea; abdominal cramps; dizziness; *photosensitivity; **kidney, *blood, and *liver disorders; rash and other allergic reactions*

Mitrofurantoin macrocrystals. See *Urogenital System*

Nafcillin sodium

Brands: Nafcil (Bristol), Unipen (Wyeth)
Capsule, Tablet, Liquid
Indication: bacterial infections
Action: treats bacterial infections
Possible side effects: nausea; vomiting; diarrhea; *rash and other allergic reactions*

Nalidixic acid   ☐ I

Brand: Neg Gram (Winthrop)
Liquid, Capsule
Indication: bacterial infections, particularly of the urinary tract
Action: treats bacterial infection
Possible side effects: nausea; vomiting; diarrhea; abdominal pain; joint pain; *photosensitivity; vision disturbances; dizziness; weakness; headache; drowsiness; *convulsions; rash and other allergic reactions*

Neomycin sulfate, hydrocortisone, acetic acid. See *Ear, Nose, and Throat*

Neomycin sulfate, polymyxin B sulfate, zinc bacitracin. See *Eyes*

Nystatin

Brands: Candex (Dome), Nilstat (Lederle)
Liquid, Ointment, Cream
Indication: fungal infections
Action: fights fungal infections
Possible side effects: irritation of the skin

Nystatin. See *Urogenital System*

Penicillin G potassium

Generic manufacturers: Squibb, Purepac, Comer, Rexall, Pfizer, Pfipharmecs, Smith Kline & French
Brand: Pentids (Squibb)
Tablet, Powder, Liquid, Injection
Indication: bacterial infections
Action: treats bacterial infections
Possible side effects: nausea; vomiting; diarrhea; dizziness; *rash and other allergic reactions*

Penicillin V potassium

Brands: Penicillin VK (Comer), Pen-Vee K (Wyeth), V-Cillin K (Lilly)

Tablet, Liquid
Indication: bacterial infections
Action: treats bacterial infections
Possible side effects: nausea; vomiting; diarrhea; dizziness; *rash and other allergic reactions*

Piperazine
Brand: Antepar (Burroughs Wellcome)
Liquid, Tablet
Indications: roundworm; pinworm
Action: treats worm infestation
Possible side effects: nausea; vomiting; diarrhea; abdominal cramps; skin discoloration; blurred vision; dizziness; headache; tremors; *convulsions; rash and other allergic reactions*

Polymyxin B, bacitracin. See *Eyes*

Polymyxin B, bacitracin, neomycin, hydrocortisone. See *Eyes*

Prednisolone acetate, sulfacetamide sodium. See *Eyes*

Pyrantel pamoate
Brand: Antiminth (Roerig)
Liquid
Indications: roundworm; pinworm
Action: treats worm infestation
Possible side effects: anorexia; nausea; vomiting; diarrhea; abdominal cramps; headache; insomnia; drowsiness; dizziness; *rash and other allergic reactions*

Pyrimethamine F
Brand: Daraprim (Burroughs Wellcome)
Tablet
Indication; parasitic infection, especially malaria
Action: treats parasitic infection
Possible side effects: anorexia; vomiting; tongue inflammation; convulsions; **blood disorders*

Quinine sulfate, aminophylline. See *Musculo-Skeletal System*

Rifampin I
Brands: Rifadin (Dow), Rimactane (CIBA)
Capsule
Indication: tuberculosis
Action: treats tubercular infection
Possible side effects: anorexia; nausea; vomiting; diarrhea; abdominal cramps; headache; dizziness; drowsiness; confusion; *vision disturbances*

Silver Nitrate. See *Eyes*

Sulfamethoxazole I
Brand: Gantanol (Roche)
Tablet, Liquid
Indication: bacterial infections
Action: treats bacterial infection
Possible side effects: anorexia; nausea; vomiting; diarrhea; joint pain; brown urine; **photosensitivity;* drowsiness; dizziness; headache; **liver, *kidney, and *blood disorders; *secondary infection; rash and other allergic reactions*

Sulfanilamide, aminacrine hydrochloride, allantoin. See *Urogenital System*

Sulfasalazine I
Brand: Azulfidine (Pharmacia)
Tablet
Indication: ulcerative colitis

Action; reduces symptoms of ulcerative colitis
Possible side effects: anorexia; nausea; vomiting; diarrhea; joint pain; brown urine; *photosensitivity; drowsiness; dizziness; headache; *liver, *kidney, and *blood disorders; *secondary infection; rash and other allergic reactions*

Sulfathiazole, sulfacetamide, sulfabenzamide. See *Urogenital System*

Sulfisoxazole. See *Urogenital System*

Sulfisoxazole diolamine. See *Eyes*

Sulfisoxazole, phenazopyridine hydrochloride. See *Urogenital System*

Tetracycline hydrochloride ☐

Generic manufacturers: Comer, Premo, Purepac, Rexall

Brands: Achromycin (Lederle), Sumycin (Squibb), Tetracyn (Pfipharmecs)

Capsule, Liquid, Injection

Indication: bacterial infections

Action: treats bacterial infections

Possible side effects: anorexia; nausea; vomiting; diarrhea; tongue inflammation; *photosensitivity; joint pain; *kidney, *liver, and *blood disorders; *superinfections; rash and other allergic reactions*

Trimethoprim, sulfamethoxazole ☐

Brands: Septra, Septra DS (Burroughs Wellcome), Bactrim, Bactrim DS (Roche)

Tablet, Liquid

Indication: bacterial infections

Action: treats bacterial infection

Possible side effects: anorexia; nausea; vomiting; diarrhea; joint pain; brown urine; *photosensitivity; drowsiness; dizziness; headache; *liver, *kidney, and *blood disorders; *secondary infection; rash and other allergic reactions*

See also listing for Sulfamethoxazole

Vancomycin hydrochloride

Brand: Vancocin (Lilly)

Liquid

Indication; bacterial infections, particularly intestinal

Action: treats bacterial infections

Possible side effects: nausea; *superinfection; rash and other allergic reactions*

Vidarabine. See *Eyes*

NONPRESCRIPTION DRUGS

Aftate (Plough)

Powder, Liquid (topical), Gel

Indication: topical fungal infections

Action: reduces fungus

Bacimycin Ointment (Merrell-National)

Ointment

Indications: minor cuts; burns; abrasions; skin irritations

Action: reduces chance of infection

Bacitracin Topical Ointment (Pfipharmecs)

Ointment

Indications: minor cuts; burns; abrasions; skin irritations

Action: reduces chance of infection

Bactine (Miles)

Aerosol, Liquid (topical)

Indication: skin wounds

Action: reduces chance of infection

Betadine Solution, Betadine Skin Cleanser (Purdue Frederick)

Liquid (topical)

Indication: prevention of skin infections

Action: reduces chance of infection

B.F.I. Antiseptic First-Aid Powder (Beecham)

Powder

Indications: cuts; abrasions; burns; scratches; prickly heat; insect bites; athlete's foot; poison ivy and oak

Actions: reduces chance of infection; relieves itching, chafing, and irritation

BPN Triple Antibiotic Ointment (Norwich-Eaton)

Ointment

Indications: minor cuts; abrasions

Action: reduces chance of infection

Campho-Phenique Liquid. See *Mouth and Teeth*

Chloraseptic. See *Mouth and Teeth*

Chloresium Ointment and Solution. See *Mouth and Teeth*

Cruex (Pharmacraft)

Powder, Cream

Indication: bacterial or fungal infection

Action: reduces bacteria and fungi

Desenex (Pharmacraft)

Powder, Ointment, Liquid (topical), Soap

Indications: athlete's foot; ringworm

Action: reduces bacteria and fungi

Fostex BPO 5%. See *Skin, Hair, and Scalp*

Isodine Antiseptic (Blair)

Liquid (topical)

Indications: minor cuts; burns; abrasions

Action: reduces chance of infection

Johnson & Johnson First Aid Cream (Johnson & Johnson)

Cream

Indications: minor burns; abrasions; cuts

Action: reduces chance of infection

Medicone Dressing Cream (Medicone)

Cream

Indications: minor burns; wounds; diaper rash; abrasions; skin irritations

Actions: reduces chance of infection; relieves pain, burning, and itching

Medi-Quik (Lehn & Fink)

Spray

Indications: sunburn; cuts; scrapes; poison ivy; burns; insect bites

Actions: reduces chance of infection; relieves pain

Mercurochrome (Becton Dickinson)

Liquid (topical)

Indications: cuts; scratches; burns; abrasions

Action: reduces chance of infection

Myciguent Antibiotic Ointment (Upjohn)

Ointment

Indications: minor cuts; burns; abrasions; skin irritations

Action: reduces chance of infection

Mycitracin Antibiotic Ointment (Upjohn)

Ointment

Indications: minor cuts; burns; abrasions; skin irritations

Action: reduces chance of infection

Norwich Bacitracin Antibiotic Ointment (Norwich-Eaton)

Ointment

Indications: minor cuts; burns; abrasions

Action: reduces chance of infection
Roma-Nol (Jamol)
Liquid (topical)
Indications: skin and mucous membrane infections
Action: reduces chance of infection
S.T. 37. See *Pain*
Terramycin Ointment (Pfipharmecs)
Ointment
Indications: minor cuts; burns; abrasions
Action: treats infection
Tinactin (Schering)
Cream, Liquid (topical), Powder, Aerosol
Indication: fungal infections, such as athlete's foot, jock itch, body ringworm
Action: treats fungal infections
Vagisil Feminine Itching Medication. See *Urogenital System*
Vanoxide Acne Lotion. See *Skin, Hair, and Scalp*

Mouth and Teeth

Infection:
The mouth and teeth are constantly exposed to "germs" such as bacteria and viruses. They are usually able to defend against infection unless some damage has occurred to the tissues, such as a cut or a cavity in the tooth. In these cases, treatment should include not only a drug to treat the infection but also a search to find the underlying cause. This cause may not be localized, but may in fact be a general problem in the body, such as anemia or diabetes, which make the body more susceptible to infection.

Pain:
Sometimes pain in the mouth or teeth is not caused by a problem in that area but instead is referred to the mouth from some other area, such as the heart or lungs. For example, some patients with angina have pain in their teeth and jaw upon physical exertion. By the same mechanism of "referred pain," problems in the teeth and mouth can cause pain elsewhere. For example, headaches may be caused by a poor bite, "malocclusion." In either case, the important message is the same: chronic pain, even if relieved by medication, deserves a medical evaluation to find the underlying cause.

Bad Breath (Halitosis):
Chronic bad breath is an indication of an underlying problem. Until that cause is determined, the individual should not simply rely on mouthwashes to counteract the bad odor. The cause may be local (gum infections, post-nasal drip from inflamed sinuses, dental cavities, etc.) or may be systemic (diabetes or leukemia).

PRESCRIPTION DRUGS

Cortisol acetate
Brand: Orabase HCA (Hoyte)
Paste
Indication: oral inflammation
Action: relieves pain and inflammation
Possible side effects: irritation; peptic ulcer
Doxycycline. See *Infection*
Erythromycin. See *Infection*

Nystatin
Brand: Nilstat (Lederle)
Liquid
Indication: oral fungal infections
Action: reduces fungus
Possible side effects: nausea; vomiting; diarrhea; abdominal cramps
Tetracycline hydrochloride. See *Infection*
Triamcinolone acetonide
Brand: Kenalog in Orabase (Squibb)
Paste
Indication: oral inflammation
Action: relieves pain and inflammation
Possible side effects: irritation; *peptic ulcer*

NONPRESCRIPTION DRUGS

Anbesol Antiseptic Anesthetic Liquid (Whitehall)
Liquid (topical)
Indications: teething; toothache; cold sores and blisters; cuts, scrapes, and burns
Actions: relieves pain; reduces infection
Blistex (Blistex)
Balm
Indications: cold sore; fever blister; chapped, dry lips; sunburn
Action: moisturizes
Campho-Phenique Liquid (Winthrop)
Liquid (topical), Gel
Indications: fever blisters; cold sores; cuts; burns; sores; insect bites
Actions: relieves pain; reduces infection
Cankaid (Becton Dickinson)
Liquid (topical)
Indications: canker sores; sore gums; denture irritation; mouth inflammation
Actions: relieves inflammation; reduces irritation
Cēpacol Anesthetic Troches (Merrell-National)
Lozenge
Indication: mouth and throat irritations and inflammation
Actions: relieves pain; reduces dryness
Cēpacol Mouthwash/Gargle. See *Ear, Nose, and Throat*
Cēpastat. See *Ear, Nose, and Throat*
Chap Stick Lip Balm (Miller-Morton)
Balm
Indication: chapped, dry lips
Actions: moisturizes; prevents sunburn
Chloraseptic, Chloraseptic Lozenges (Norwich-Eaton)
Liquid (topical), Spray, Lozenge
Indications: throat, mouth, and gum irritations and inflammation
Actions: relieves pain and inflammation; reduces infection; deodorizes
Chloraseptic Children's Lozenges. See *Ear, Nose, and Throat*
Chloraseptic Gel (Norwich-Eaton)
Gel
Indication: mouth and gum irritations
Action: relieves pain
Chloresium Ointment and Solution (Rystan)
Ointment, Liquid (topical)
Indications: pain, inflammation, and odor in cuts, burns,

abrasions, and skin irritations

Actions: relieves pain and inflammation; reduces odor

Cushion Grip (Plough)

Soft adhesive

Indication: adhesive for plastic and porcelain dentures

Action: secures dentures

Dalidyne (Dalin)

Liquid (topical)

Indications: fever blisters; canker sores; teething pain; herpes simplex; mouth, throat, denture, and gum inflammation and irritations

Actions: soothes; reduces infection

Derma Medicone (Medicone)

Ointment

Indications: oral and denture irritation; insect bites; eczema; prickly heat; sunburn

Actions: reduces irritation; relieves pain

Fluorigard Anti-Cavity Dental Rinse (Colgate-Palmolive)

Liquid (topical)

Indication: cavity prevention

Action: reduces cavities

Gly-Oxide Liquid (Marion)

Liquid (topical)

Indications: canker sores; denture irritation

Action: reduces irritation

Listerine Antiseptic (Warner-Lambert)

Liquid

Indications: mouth and throat irritations; oral rinse; minor cuts; insect bites; dandruff

Actions: reduces irritation and infection; refreshes mouth

Mersene Denture Cleanser (Colgate-Palmolive)

Powder

Indication: denture cleaning

Action: cleans dentures

Orabase Plain (Hoyt)

Paste

Indication: mouth and gum irritations

Actions: soothes; reduces irritation

Orabase with Benzocaine (Hoyt)

Paste

Indication: mouth and gum irritations

Action: relieves pain; reduces irritation

Protect Toothpaste (Marion)

Paste

Indication: cleaning of sensitive teeth

Action: cleans and protects sensitive teeth

Proxigel (Reed & Carnrick)

Gel

Indications: oral inflammation; canker sores

Actions: soothes; reduces infection

Scope (Proctor & Gamble)

Liquid (topical)

Indications: mouth and throat irritations; oral rinse

Actions: refreshes mouth; reduces mouth and throat irritations

Sensodyne Toothpaste (Block)

Paste

Indication: cleaning of sensitive teeth

Action: cleans and protects sensitive teeth

S.T. 37 (Beecham)

Liquid (topical)

Indications: burns; cuts; abrasions; sunburn; mouth irritations

Actions: relieves pain; reduces irritation and infection

Vaseline Constant Care (Chesebrough Ponds)
Balm

Indication: chapped, dry lips

Action: moisturizes

Musculo-Skeletal System

The musculo-skeletal system includes the body's muscles, bones, ligaments, tendons, and joints. The most common problems in this system are muscle aches and soreness. Arthritis and gout are two disorders that affect the joints.

MUSCLE ACHES AND SORENESS

Muscle aches and soreness are usually caused by unusual strain on the muscle from exercise, emotional tension, or jarring moves. When this occurs, muscle fibers may tear and cause slight bleeding into the muscle ("black and blue marks").

Ice and Heat. The muscle tearing leads to pain, inflammation, and spasm. If ice is applied immediately after the injury, the localized blood vessels constrict and the bleeding and resultant inflammation are reduced. If heat is applied hours after the injury, circulation to the area is increased, which soothes the pain, helps break the spasm, and speeds up the reabsorption of irritating substances. Ice and heat used in this way will enhance the effect of the medication.

Muscle Pain. Most prescription and nonprescription drugs taken by mouth to treat muscle pain combine the same ingredients as those drugs listed in the Pain section. Although drugs applied topically may have a soothing action and thereby secondarily relieve the pain, they are not specifically "muscle pain killers."

Muscle Inflammation. The irritation of the torn muscle fibers and bleeding causes inflammatory redness and swelling. Steroids such as cortisone can be taken orally or given locally by injection for this problem, if the potential benefits outweigh the risk. The inflammation often will respond to time and other drugs, such as aspirin and local ointments or lotions.

Muscle Spasm. Sometimes the afflicted person cannot recall any overuse or incident that might have caused the muscle spasm. This is particularly true for spasm in the neck or lower back muscles. In such cases the spasm is often caused by emotional tension or weakness or injury to other muscles in the area. The muscles in spasm—"stiff as boards"—are actually trying to protect and support adjacent weak muscles and are over-compensating. Drugs used to break the spasm will be most effective if the underlying cause is determined and treated so that the protective spasm is no longer necessary.

ARTHRITIS AND GOUT

Arthritis is inflammation of the joints. The most common form is osteoarthritis, which in some people occurs with the wear and tear of aging and causes pain and stiffness in many joints throughout the body. Pain medications, such as aspirin, not only reduce the discomfort and inflammation, but they also enable the individual to move the joint, which in itself is therapeutic. If the afflicted joints remain immobile, calcium deposits around the joints cause additional stiffness and soreness. Rheumatoid arthritis is caused by an allergic inflammatory process at specific joints, particularly the middle finger joints. Along with drugs for the pain, medicines such as steroids are also prescribed to reduce the allergic reaction. Gout is caused by an unusual increase in one of the blood's necessary components, uric acid. This excess acid may crystallize and cause kidney stones or the acid may irritate joints, particularly the big toes. Drugs are used to reduce the uric acid levels and to relieve the pain and decrease the swelling when flareups occur. Finally, when arthritis is caused by an infection in the joint, such as gonorrhea, antibiotics are prescribed.

Muscle Aches

PRESCRIPTION DRUGS

Acetaminophen, chlorzoxazone [I]
Brand: Parafon Forte (McNeil)
Tablet
Indication: muscle and joint pain
Actions: relaxes muscles; relieves pain
Possible side effects: nausea; indigestion; lightheadedness; drowsiness; urine discoloration; *rash and other allergic reactions*
See also listing for Chlorzoxazone

Aspirin, caffeine, orphenadrine citrate, phenacetin [D] [I]
Brand: Norgesic, Norgesic Forte (Riker)
Tablet
Indication: muscle and joint pain
Action: relieves pain
Possible side effects: nausea; vomiting; constipation; dry mouth; nasal congestion; dizziness; headache; lightheadedness; blurred vision; agitation; *urinary difficulties; rash and other allergic reactions*

Baclofen [D] [I]
Brand: Lioresal (Geigy)
Tablet
Indication: muscle spasm
Actions: relaxes muscles; relieves spasticity
Possible side effects: anorexia; nausea; vomiting; diarrhea; constipation; *urinary difficulties; impotence; nasal congestion; drowsiness; dizziness; headache; *rash and other allergic reactions*

Betamethasone. See *Cancer*

Betamethasone valerate. See *Skin, Hair, and Scalp*

Carisoprodol [D] [I]
Brand: Soma (Wallace)
Tablet
Indication: muscle spasm
Actions: relaxes muscles; relieves pain
Possible side effects: nausea; vomiting; constipation; nervousness; drowsiness; headache; blurred vision; *rash and other allergic reactions*

Chlorzoxazone [I]
Brand: Paraflex (McNeil)
Tablet

Indication: muscle spasm
Action: relaxes muscles
Possible side effects: nausea; indigestion and intestinal irritation; urine discoloration; drowsiness; dizziness; lightheadedness; nervousness; *abnormal bruising; rash and other allergic reactions*

Cyclobenzaprine hydrochloride [I]
Brand: Flexeril (Merck Sharp & Dohme)
Tablet
Indication: muscle spasm
Action: relaxes muscles
Possible side effects: nausea; constipation; dry mouth; drowsiness; fatigue; blurred vision; insomnia; dizziness; headache; euphoria; weakness; urinary retention; increased perspiring; palpitations; *rash and other allergic reactions*

Fluocinolone acetonide. See *Skin, Hair, and Scalp*
Fluocinonide. See *Skin, Hair, and Scalp*
Flurandrenolide. See *Skin, Hair, and Scalp*
Iodochlorhydroxyquin, hydrocortisone. See *Skin, Hair, and Scalp*

Metaxalone
Brand: Skelaxin (Robins)
Tablet
Indication: musculo-skeletal pain and spasm
Actions: relieves pain; sedates
Possible side effects: nausea; vomiting; abdominal cramps; nervousness; drowsiness; headache; dizziness; *decrease in white and red blood cells; rash and other allergic reactions*

Methocarbamol [I]
Brand: Robaxin, Robaxin-750 (Robins)
Tablet
Indication: musculo-skeletal spasm
Action: relaxes muscles
Possible side effects: nausea; lightheadedness; dizziness; drowsiness; headache; blurred vision; nasal congestion; urine discoloration; *rash and other allergic reactions*

Nystatin, neomycin sulfate, gramicidin, triamcinolone acetonide. See *Skin, Hair, and Scalp*

Orphenadrine citrate [I]
Brand: Norflex (Riker)
Tablet
Indication: muscle strain
Actions: relieves pain; sedates
Possible side effects: nausea; vomiting; constipation; dry mouth; blurred vision; *urinary difficulties; drowsiness; lightheadedness; weakness; headache; nervousness; palpitations; rash and other allergic reactions*

Quinine sulfate, aminophylline
Brand: Quinamm (Merrell-National)
Tablet
Indication: muscle cramps
Action: relaxes muscles
Possible side effects: nausea; vomiting; abdominal cramps; diarrhea; nervousness; ringing in ears; dizziness; confusion; headache; *palpitations; rash and other allergic reactions*

Triamcinolone acetonide. See *Skin, Hair, and Scalp*
Zomepirac sodium. See *Pain*

NONPRESCRIPTION DRUGS

Bayer Aspirin. See *Pain*
Bayer Timed-Release Aspirin. See *Pain*
Ben-Gay External Analgesic (Leeming)
Ointment, Lotion, Gel
Indication: pain in muscles and joints
Action: relieves pain
DeWitt's Pills for Backache and Joint Pains (DeWitt)
Tablet
Indications: backache and joint pain; muscle aches; head-
    aches
Action: relieves pain
Goody's Headache Powders. See *Nervous System*
Icy Hot (Searle)
Balm
Indication: muscle pain
Action: relieves pain
InfraRub Analgesic (Whitehall)
Cream
Indication: muscle, joint, and nerve pain
Action: relieves pain
Momentum (Whitehall)
Tablet
Indication: muscular backache
Action: relieves pain and inflammation
Myoflex Creme (Warren-Teed)
Cream
Indication: muscle and joint pain
Action: relieves pain and stiffness
Stanback Analgesic Powders (Stanback)
Powder
Indications: neuralgia; muscle aches and pains; arthritis;
    headaches; fever; menstrual discomfort
Actions: reduces inflammation and fever; relieves pain

Arthritis

PRESCRIPTION DRUGS

Dexamethasone
Generic manufacturers: Purepac, Smith Kline & French
Brand: Decadron (Merck Sharp & Dohme)
Liquid, Tablet
Indications: arthritis; bursitis; gout; psoriasis; endocrine
    disorders; allergy; colitis; cancer
Action: reduces inflammation
Possible side effects: indigestion; appetite changes; dizzi-
    ness; headache; weakness; weight gain; abnormal hair
    growth; emotional disturbances; fluid retention; muscle
    cramps; acne; menstrual changes; *aggravation of poten-
    tial heart or ulcer problem; increased blood pressure; in-
    flammation of pancreas; rash and other allergic reactions*
Fenoprofen calcium   F
Brand: Nalfon (Dista)
Capsule
Indication: arthritis
Actions: reduces inflammation and fever; relieves pain
Possible side effects: anorexia; nausea; vomiting; diarrhea;
    abdominal cramps; dry mouth; drowsiness; nervousness
    or depression; palpitations; loss of hair; vision disturb-
    ances; *kidney, *blood, and *liver disorders; rash and
    other allergic reactions*

Fludrecortisone acetate. See *Hormones*

Hydrocortisone

Brands: Cortef (Upjohn), Cortenema (Rowell), Cortril (Pfi-pharmecs), Hydrocortone (Merck Sharp & Dohme)

Tablet, Liquid, Suppository, Cream, Gel, Spray

Indication: inflammation

Action: reduces inflammation

Possible side effects: indigestion; appetite changes; weight gain; acne; rash; abnormal hair growth; emotional disturbances; fluid retention; headache; dizziness; muscle cramps; menstrual changes; reactivated tuberculosis; *aggravation of potential heart or ulcer problem; increased blood pressure; inflamed pancreas*

Ibuprofen [F]

Brand: Motrin (Upjohn)

Tablet

Indication: arthritis

Actions: reduces inflammation and fever; relieves pain

Possible side effects: anorexia; nausea; diarrhea; abdominal cramps; vision disturbances; ringing in ears; dizziness; lightheadedness; headache; fluid retention; weight gain; nervousness; *blood and *liver disorders; stomach irritation and bleeding; rash and other allergic reactions*

Indomethacin [F]

Brand: Indocin (Merck Sharp & Dohme)

Capsule

Indications: arthritis; inflammation, especially of joints

Actions: reduces inflammation and fever; relieves pain

Possible side effects: anorexia; nausea; vomiting; diarrhea; abdominal cramps; lightheadedness; dizziness; ringing in ears; fluid retention; breast enlargement; headache; drowsiness; emotional disturbances; loss of hair; *urinary difficulties; stomach irritation and bleeding; *blood and *liver disorders; rash and other allergic reactions*

Note: take with an antacid

Methylprednisolone

Brand: Medrol (Oral) (Upjohn)

Tablet

Indication: inflammation

Action: reduces inflammation

Possible side effects: indigestion; appetite changes; weight gain; acne; rash; abnormal hair growth; emotional disturbances; fluid retention; headache; dizziness; muscle cramps; menstrual changes; reactivated tuberculosis; *aggravation of potential heart or ulcer problem; increased blood pressure; inflamed pancreas*

Naproxen [F]

Brand: Naprosyn (Syntex)

Tablet

Indication: arthritis

Actions: reduces inflammation and fever; relieves pain

Possible side effects: nausea; vomiting; indigestion; abdominal cramps; diarrhea; constipation; lightheadedness; drowsiness; dizziness; headache; ringing in ears; fluid retention; increased perspiring; palpitations; *gastrointestinal bleeding; *liver and *kidney disorders; rash and other allergic reactions*

Oxyphenbutazone [F]

Brands: Oxalid (USV),Tandearil (Geigy)

Tablet

Indications: arthritis; gout; inflammation

Actions: reduces inflammation and fever; relieves pain

Possible side effects: nausea; vomiting; heartburn; diarrhea; constipation; drowsiness; agitation; confusion; tremors; headache; weakness; ringing in ears; fluid retention; increased blood pressure; *gastrointestinal bleeding; *liver, *kidney, and *blood disorders; rash and other allergic reactions*

Note: take with milk

Penicillamine

Brands: Cuprimine (Merck Sharp & Dohme), Depen Titratabs (Wallace)

Capsule, Tablet

Indications: rheumatoid arthritis; lead poisoning; copper metabolism disorders

Actions: eliminates toxic metals from body; relieves severe arthritis

Possible side effects: anorexia; nausea; vomiting; diarrhea; loss of taste; joint and muscle pain; ringing in ears; headache; ulcers in mouth; *blood and *kidney disorders; rash and other allergic reactions*

Phenylbutazone   F

Brand: Butazolidin (Geigy)

Tablet, Capsule

Indications: arthritis; gout; inflammation, especially of the joints

Actions: reduces inflammation and fever; relieves pain

Possible side effects: nausea; indigestion; diarrhea; constipation; drowsiness; agitation; confusion; tremors; headache; weakness; fluid retention; increased blood pressure; *gastrointestinal bleeding; *kidney, *liver, and *blood disorders; rash and other allergic reactions*

Phenylbutazone, dried aluminum hydroxide gel, magnesium trisilicate   F

Brand: Butazolidin Alka (Geigy)

Tablet, Capsule

Indications: arthritis; gout; inflammation

Actions: reduces inflammation and fever; relieves pain

Possible side effects: nausea; indigestion; diarrhea; constipation; drowsiness; agitation; confusion; tremors; headache; weakness; fluid retention; increased blood pressure; *gastrointestinal bleeding; *kidney, *liver, and *blood disorders; rash and other allergic reactions*

See also listing for Phenylbutazone

Prednisone Oral   P

Generic manufacturers: American Pharmaceutical, Comer, Philips Roxane, Premo, Purepac, Rexall

Brands: Deltasone (Upjohn), Meticorten (Schering), Paracort (Parke-Davis)

Tablet

Indication: inflammation

Action: reduces inflammation

Possible side effects: indigestion; appetite changes; weight gain; acne; rash; abnormal hair growth; emotional disturbances; fluid retention; headache; dizziness; muscle cramps; menstrual changes; reactivated tuberculosis; *aggravation of potential heart or ulcer problem; increased blood pressure; inflamed pancreas*

Note: restrict salt; take with a protein-rich diet

Sulindac   F

Brand: Clinoril (Merck Sharp & Dohme)
Tablet
Indication: arthritis
Actions: reduces inflammation and fever; relieves pain
Possible side effects: nausea; indigestion; vomiting; constipation; blurred vision; ringing in ears; drowsiness; confusion; dizziness; numbness; tingling; headache; fluid retention; *intestinal bleeding; *bone marrow depression; rash and other allergic reactions*

Tolmetin sodium
Brands: Tolectin, Tolectin DS (McNeil)
Tablet
Indication: arthritis
Actions: reduces inflammation and fever; relieves pain
Possible side effects: nausea; indigestion; vomiting; abdominal cramps; diarrhea; constipation; nervousness; drowsiness; lightheadedness; ringing in ears; dizziness; headache; fluid retention; increased blood pressure; *intestinal bleeding; *bone marrow depression; rash and other allergic reactions*
Note: take 1—2 hours after eating, with antacids or some food

Triamcinolone
Brand: Aristocort (Lederle)
Tablet, Liquid
Indication: inflammation
Action: reduces inflammation
Possible side effects: anorexia; drowsiness; dizziness; vertigo; headache; flushing; fluid retention; muscle weakness; mental changes; skin discoloration; increased sweating; menstrual changes; increased blood pressure; *increased eye pressure; increased risk of bone fractures; gastric bleeding; cataracts*

NONPRESCRIPTION DRUGS

Arthritis Pain Formula (Whitehall)
Tablet
Indications: arthritis; pain; fever
Actions: relieves pain; reduces fever and inflammation
Ascriptin (Rorer)
Tablet
Indications: arthritis; headache; neuralgia; menstrual cramps; cold; flu
Actions: reduces inflammation and fever; relieves pain
Ascriptin A/D Arthritis Doses (Rorer)
Tablet
Indication: arthritis
Actions: relieves pain; reduces fever and inflammation
Aspercreme (Thompson)
Lotion, Cream
Indications: arthritis; muscular aches; burning and tingling of hands and feet
Action: relieves pain
Arthritis Strength Bufferin (Bristol-Myers)
Tablet
Indications: arthritis; pain; fever
Actions: relieves pain; reduces fever and inflammation
Aspirin Suppositories. See *Pain*

Cama Inlay-Tabs (Dorsey)
Tablet
Indications: arthritis; rheumatism
Action: relieves pain
Deep-Down (Williams)
Ointment
Indications: arthritis; muscle aches; backache
Action: relieves pain
Ecotrin (Menley & James)
Tablet
Indication: arthritis
Action: relieves pain
Heet Analgesic (Whitehall)
Liquid (topical), Spray
Indications: arthritis; neuralgia; muscle aches
Actions: relieves pain; increases blood flow to affected area
Os-Cal-Gesic (Marion)
Tablet
Indication: arthritis
Action: relieves pain
Vanquish (Glenbrook)
Capsule
Indications: arthritis; headache; muscle aches and pains;
neuralgia; cold; flu; fever; menstrual cramps
Actions: relieves pain; reduces fever

Gout

PRESCRIPTION DRUGS

Allopurinol
Brand: Zyloprim (Burroughs Wellcome)
Tablet
Indications: gout and uric acid disturbances
Action: normalizes uric acid level
Possible side effects: nausea; vomiting; diarrhea; abdominal
cramps; initial increase in attacks of gout; drowsiness;
headache; loss of hair; *kidney, nerve, or *liver
disorders; *bone marrow depression; rash and other
allergic reactions*
Colchicine
Generic manufacturers: Lilly, Purepac
Tablet, Injection
Indication: gout
Actions: reduces inflammation; relieves pain
Possible side effects: nausea; vomiting; diarrhea; abdominal
pain; loss of hair; weakness; tingling and numbness in
hands and feet; *dehydration; *bone marrow depression;
*liver, *kidney, nerve, or colon disorders; rash and other
allergic reactions*
Probenecid
Brand: Benemid (Merck Sharp & Dohme)
Tablet
Indication: gout
Action: decreases gout attacks by normalizing uric acid
level
Possible side effects: anorexia; nausea; vomiting; dizziness;
flushing; headache; weakness; kidney stones; *liver and
*kidney disorders; *bone marrow depression; rash and
other allergic reactions*

Nervous System

All medications that treat a *specific* neurological or emotional problem have a *general* effect on the nervous system, often including an effect on alertness, thinking, and mood. Any mental changes noted by you or others—drowsiness, confusion, irritability, nervousness, depression—may be attributable to these drugs. Furthermore, because the skin and gastrointestinal system are related to the nervous system, most of the following drugs commonly cause some digestive changes or skin sensitivity.

Epilepsy

Epilepsy is not just one condition; it has many different causes and manifestations. It may involve convulsions or seizures that vary from minor tics or forgetfulness to severe spasms of the entire body and complete loss of consciousness. Because epilepsy has so many different forms and because convulsions can be triggered by many different situations (such as alcohol or fatigue), the doctor and patient must work closely together to find the best drug or combination of drugs and the best dosages depending on the individual's lifestyle and tolerance of side effects.

PRESCRIPTION DRUGS

Acetazolamide. See *Cardiovascular System*

Carbamazepine [F] [I]
Brand: Tegretol (Geigy)
Tablet
Indications: seizures unresponsive to less toxic anti-convulsants; trigeminal neuralgia (a kind of facial pain)
Actions: prevents convulsions; relieves pain of trigeminal neuralgia
Possible side effects: anorexia; nausea; vomiting; diarrhea; constipation; abdominal cramps; drowsiness; dizziness; confusion; depression; fluid retention; urinary frequency; muscle and joint aches; **blood and *liver disorders; rash and other allergic reactions*

Phenobarbital [D] [I]
Generic manufacturers: Comatic, Purepac, Rexall
Tablet, Liquid
Indication: seizures
Action: reduces occurrence of seizures
Possible side effects: nausea; drowsiness; dizziness; confusion; excitement; delirium; *rash and other allergic reactions*

Phenytoin sodium [F] [I]
Brand: Dilantin (Parke-Davis)
Capsule, Tablet, Liquid, Injection
Indication: seizures
Action: reduces occurrence of seizures
Possible side effects: nausea; vomiting; constipation; dizziness; confusion; slurred speech; headache; dark urine; gum enlargement; abnormal hair growth; **blood, *liver, and heart disorders; rash and other allergic reactions*

Primidone [I]
Brand: Mysoline (Ayerst)
Tablet, Liquid
Indication: seizures
Action: reduces occurrence of seizures

Possible side effects: anorexia; nausea; vomiting; drowsiness; decreased balance and coordination; dizziness; emotional disturbances; impotence; *anemia; rash and other allergic reactions*

Headaches

The brain itself does not have pain sensation. The pain of a headache is caused by tension or pressure in the blood vessels, muscles, or sinuses in the head, scalp, or neck. Most headache remedies therefore do not work "in the brain" but simply relieve the pain in the surrounding tissues. The essential ingredient in most nonprescription medicine for headaches is simply aspirin—a pain medicine. Acetaminophen is

Headaches

Type	Character	Treatment
Tension	most common type; tension of muscles along back of neck and around scalp; occur some hours after awakening; "tight band" around head	aspirin; nonprescription headache-relief medicines
Migraine	begin with queasy feeling in stomach, or flashing lights, or blind spots; followed minutes later by pounding in one side of head; nausea, vomiting, sensitivity to noise and bright light	aspirin; antidepressants; blood vessel constrictors
Facial Pain	excruciating pain; localized; one sensitive area of face; irritated by light touch or even breeze	pain relievers; Tegretol
Sinus	behind eyes; worse in a.m.; stuffed-up feeling; post-nasal drip	pain medicine; decongestants
Temporal Arthritis	beside one eye on temple; watery eye; pounding pain; onset in late adulthood	pain relievers; anti-inflammatory drugs (corticosteroids)
Brain Tumor	persistent pain; nausea and vomiting; awakening in night	pain relievers; radiation and/or surgery

another pain medicine, preferred by those who find aspirin too irritating for their stomachs. Other ingredients, such as caffeine, are often combined with either aspirin or acetaminophen, and buffering agents are also added. The necessity of these additional ingredients for most people is controversial. Chronic headaches unrelieved by aspirin or acetaminophen and associated with nausea, vomiting, sensitivity to light, awakening from sleep, or mental changes require medical evaluation.

PRESCRIPTION DRUGS

Aspirin, phenacetin, caffeine, codeine phosphate. See *Pain*
Butalbital, aspirin, phenacetin, caffeine ⬛D ⬛I
Brand: Fiorinal (Sandoz)
Tablet, Capsule
Indication: headache
Actions: relieves pain; reduces tension
Possible side effects: nausea; vomiting; drowsiness; confusion; lightheadedness; dizziness; *rash and other allergic reactions*
Butalbital, aspirin, phenacetin, caffeine, codeine ⬛D ⬛I
Brand: Fiorinal with Codeine (Sandoz)
Capsule
Indication: headache
Actions: relieves pain; reduces tension
Possible side effects: nausea; vomiting; constipation; drowsiness; confusion; lightheadedness; dizziness; eye pupil constriction; *rash and other allergic reactions*
Codeine phosphate, acetaminophen. See *Pain*
Cyproheptadine hydrochloride. See *Allergies*
Dihydrocodeine, promethazine hydrochloride, aspirin, phenacetin, caffeine. See *Pain*
Diphenhydramine hydrochloride. See *Allergies*
Meprobamate, ethoheptazine citrate, aspirin ⬛D ⬛I
Brand: Equagesic (Wyeth)
Tablet
Actions:: relieves pain; reduces tension
Possible side effects: nausea; vomiting; drowsiness; dizziness; diminished coordination; blurred vision; **bone marrow depression; rash and other allergic reactions*
Methysergide maleate ⬛F
Brand: Sansert (Sandoz)
Tablet
Indication: migraine and other vascular headaches
Action: reduces frequency and intensity of migraine
Possible side effects: nausea; vomiting; heartburn; diarrhea; drowsiness; insomnia; lightheadedness; fluid retention; weight gain
Oxycodone hydrochloride, oxycodone terephthalate, aspirin, phenacetin, caffeine. See *Pain*
Propoxyphene hydrochloride. See *Pain*
Propoxyphene hydrochloride, aspirin, phenacetin, caffeine. See *Pain*
Propoxyphene napsylate, acetaminophen. See *Pain*
Propranolol hydrochloride. See *Cardiovascular System*

NONPRESCRIPTION DRUGS

Anacin. See *Pain*
Aspirin Suppositories. See *Pain*
Bayer Aspirin. See *Pain*

Bufferin. See *Pain*
Coricidin Sinus Headache Tablets. See *Ear, Nose, and Throat*
Datril 500. See *Pain*
Excedrin. See *Pain*
Goody's Headache Powders (Goody's)
Powder
Indications: pain; headache; muscle aches; cold; fever
Actions: relieves pain; reduces fever and inflammation
Novahistine Sinus Tablets. See *Allergies*
Oraphen-PD (Additive Free). See *Pain*
Sinarest Tablets. See *Allergies*
Sine-Aid Sinus Headache Tablets. See *Ear, Nose, and Throat*
Sine-Off AF Aspirin-Free Extra Strength Tablets. See *Allergies*
Sine-Off Tablets-Aspirin Formula. See *Allergies*
Sinutab Extra Strength. See *Allergies*
Sinutab Tablets. See *Allergies*
Sinutab-II Tablets. See *Ear, Nose, and Throat*
Tylenol. See *Pain*

Parkinsonism

Parkinsonism varies widely in its symptoms and progression but generally is characterized by a tremor, a flat expression, a stooped posture, and a halting speech. The tremor becomes worse with tension or at rest and disappears with sleep. Medication can be helpful in reducing the tremor and rigidity but should be combined with speech therapy and maintaining ordinary activities when feasible. The medicines for Parkinsonism often cause mental changes that must be distinguished from the disease itself. Also, adjustment of dosages is required as the illness progresses.

PRESCRIPTION DRUGS

Amantadine hydrochloride [1]
Brand: Symmetrel (Endo)
Capsule, Liquid
Indications: Parkinsonism; tremors
Action: reduces abnormal movements caused by drugs or disease
Possible side effects: anorexia; nausea; vomiting; constipation; dry mouth; insomnia; confusion; dizziness; vision disturbances; depression; fluid retention; emotional disturbances; urinary retention; *rash and other allergic reactions*

Benztropine mesylate
Brand: Cogentin (Merck Sharp & Dohme)
Tablet, Injection
Indications: Parkinsonism; tremors
Action: reduces abnormal movements caused by drugs or disease
Possible side effects: nausea; vomiting; constipation; dry mouth; nervousness; confusion; lightheadedness; blurred vision; depression; sensitivity of eyes to strong light; urinary hesitancy; *rash and other allergic reactions*

Diphenhydramine hydrochloride. See *Allergies*

Levodopa
Generic manufacturer: Steri-Med
Capsule

Indications: Parkinsonism; tremors

Action: reduces abnormal movements caused by drugs or disease

Possible side effects: anorexia; nausea; vomiting; diarrhea; constipation; dry mouth; dizziness; blurred vision; insomnia; headache; depression; fluid retention; emotional disturbances; palpitations; *rash and other allergic reactions*

Trihexyphenidyl hydrochloride   D

Brand: Artane (Lederle)

Tablet, Capsule, Liquid

Indications: Parkinsonism; tremors

Action: reduces abnormal movements caused by drugs or disease

Possible side effects: nausea; vomiting; constipation; dry mouth; confusion; lightheadedness; blurred vision; nervousness; emotional disturbances; sensitivity of the eyes to strong light; urinary hesitancy or retention; *rash and other allergic reactions*

The Mind

Medications for the mind, called psychotropic medications, treat the symptoms associated with emotional problems. The drugs alone are not sufficient to treat chronic mental disorders, which require various kinds of psychotherapy as well. The continuous unsupervised use of psychotropic medication is ill-advised and may lead to physical or psychological dependence. In addition, many of these drugs can cause anxiety, agitation, tremulousness, irritability, seizures, and even death when stopped abruptly. If psychotropic medications have been taken for several weeks, the dosage should be decreased gradually over a period of days or even weeks when medication is no longer needed. Finally, the required dosages vary widely from individual to individual. The doctor and patient must work closely together over time to find the dosage with the best therapeutic effect and the fewest side effects. Such experimentation is usually unavoidable with this group of drugs.

Major Tranquilizers. Major tranquilizers help diminish the symptoms of severe emotional disorders, including hearing or seeing imaginary things (hallucinations), being unusually suspicious and withdrawn (paranoia), having trouble organizing thoughts, or feeling overwhelming panic. Unfortunately, some chronic psychiatric illnesses require that these medications be taken continuously and, as a result, the individual may be more susceptible to a movement disorder, which may be irreversible and untreatable. These drugs should therefore be used only when clearly indicated. However, most side effects of these drugs are temporary, reversible, or treatable. Some patients become depressed or restless with these tranquilizers; these side effects from the drug must be distinguished from the underlying psychiatric or physical disorder causing the emotional symptoms.

Mild Tranquilizers. Mild tranquilizers diminish anxiety and the associated physical discomfort such as tightness in the chest, shortness of breath, nausea, queasiness, palpitations, profuse perspiring, and tense muscles. This kind of apprehension and distress may be a symptom of a physical or emotional disorder requiring medical evaluation and treatment. However, most anxiety is normal, is an unavoidable aspect of life, and does *not* require medication. In fact, anxiety—even though disquieting—may enhance performance. Mild tranquilizers are therefore indicated for those occasions when an individual temporarily feels so overwhelmed that the usual coping mechanisms cannot work adaptively. Finally, although these tranquilizers are the most commonly prescribed and used drugs in the United States, they have serious risks, including confusion, depression, and psychological and physical dependence. They should not be used casually or continuously.

Anti-depressants. The emotional symptoms of depression include feeling suicidal, worthless, guilty, hopeless, helpless, empty, and frightened of the future or of losing one's mind. The behavioral symptoms include social withdrawal, agitation, or retarded movements. The physical symptoms include constipation, dry mouth, fatigue, change in sleep pattern, and loss of appetite, weight, and libido. These clusters of symptoms must be distinguished from grief, which is the normal sadness associated with life's unavoidable losses. Unlike grief, depression may require medical treatment.

Anti-depressant drugs rarely have an immediate effect in lifting one's mood. Although the associated anxiety and sleeplessness may improve the first couple of days, the depression itself may not be completely resolved until the drug has been taken in effectively high dosages for a few weeks. Patience and medical attention are necessary during this time. The common side effects, such as drowsiness, blurred vision, dry mouth, urinary difficulties, and constipation, either are temporary or can be relieved after consulting a doctor. Some individuals, however, because of the underlying depression, may become preoccupied with these annoying side effects, fear a severe consequence of taking the drug, and stop the medication prematurely.

Mood Stabilizers. Lithium is a salt that has been helpful in reducing the frequency and severity of manic episodes, which are characterized by feelings of elation, grandiose ideas, limited sleep requirements, and often unreasonable plans with a belligerent refusal to accept advice from others. The drug has also been used to treat the actual manic episode and may be helpful in reducing the severity and frequency of associated recurrent depressions. However, lithium has not been found helpful in treating depression. Instead, the drug has been more helpful in stabilizing the mood of individuals prone to wide swings between euphoria and despair.

Before taking the drug, the individual should have a careful evaluation to make sure of the psychiatric indications and to check the thyroid, heart, and kidneys with a physical examination, cardiogram, and blood tests. While taking the drug, the dosage must be *very carefully* adjusted. Too little is completely ineffective; too much can cause tremulousness, confusion, coma, and death. Regular blood tests to check the drug level are crucial.

Sleep medication. Sleep medication should be used only for occasional insomnia. Persistent insomnia may be a sign of a serious illness, such as hyperthyroidism or depression, and requires medical evaluation. If used nightly on a continuous basis, sleep medications tend to lose their effectiveness, require higher and higher dosages, and lead to physical and psychological dependence. Furthermore, if some sleep medications are taken nightly for several days or weeks and then discontinued, the individual may have a "rebound" effect characterized by insomnia, anxiety, restlessness, and nightmares.

When taken in high dosages or when combined with alcohol, sleep medications can cause confusion. This confusion may in turn make the individual unaware of how many pills have already been taken and lead to a fatal overdosage. Alcohol can be a poor drug for sleep. Although the individual may feel more relaxed and able to fall asleep, the depressed effect of the drug may last only two or three hours and can cause early morning awakening and depression that makes the insomnia worse. Bedwetting, nightmares, and night terrors generally should not be treated by nonprescription sleep medication. If persistent, they require medical evaluation and possibly other kinds of drugs.

Anti-sleep medication. Drugs that impede drowsiness or sleep may be helpful on isolated occasions, such as unavoidable long drives at night. These drugs stimulate the nervous system and may cause irritability and nervousness. If used continuously, they tend to be less effective, can cause personality change, and may lead to abuse and dependence. Narcolepsy is a relatively rare sleep disorder characterized by sudden sleep attacks, momentary paralysis upon awakening, sudden unanticipated collapses during the day, and strange hallucinatory sensations when falling asleep. This disorder is one of the few indications for continuing high dosages of prescription anti-sleep medication, but careful evaluation by a doctor is advised.

PRESCRIPTION DRUGS

Amitriptyline hydrochloride [I]
Brand: Elavil (Merck Sharp & Dohme)
Tablet, Injection
Indication: depression
Action: relieves depression
Possible side effects: constipation; dry mouth; lightheadedness; drowsiness; blurred vision; dizziness; tremors; impotence; *urinary difficulties; palpitations; hallucinations; *heart, *blood, and *liver disorders; rash and other allergic reactions*

Amitriptyline hydrochloride, perphenazine [I]
Brand: Triavil (Merck Sharp & Dohme)
Tablet
Indications: combination of anxiety and depression
Actions: reduces agitation; relieves depression
Possible side effects: nausea; indigestion; constipation; dry mouth; lightheadedness; drowsiness; restlessness; tremors; breast enlargement; *urinary difficulties; impotence; retarded ejaculation; *photosensitivity; menstrual changes; aggravation of diabetes; *involuntary movements of face, jaw, tongue, and mouth; palpitations; hallucinations; *blood, *heart, and *liver disorders; rash and other allergic reactions*
See also listings for Amitriptyline hydrochloride and Perphenazine

Chlorazepate dipotassium [D] [I]
Brand: Tranxene (Abbott)

Capsule
Indications: anxiety; nervous tension; alcoholic withdrawal
Action: tranquilizes
Possible side effects: dry mouth; drowsiness; nervousness; confusion; dizziness; blurred vision; insomnia; headache; fluid retention; menstrual changes; *rash and other allergic reactions*

Chlordiazepoxide hydrochloride [D] [I]
Brand: Librium (Roche)
Capsule, Tablet
Indications: anxiety; nervous tension; alcoholic withdrawal
Action: tranquilizes
Possible side effects: nausea; constipation; drowsiness; confusion; excitement; hallucinations; blurred vision; fluid retention; menstrual changes; *jaundice; rash and other allergic reactions*

Chlorpromazine [I]
Brand: Thorazine (Smith Kline & French)
Tablet
Indications: psychosis; severe anxiety; depression; hyperactivity in children
Actions: tranquilizes; reduces anxiety and associated depression; inhibits psychomotor functions
Possible side effects: constipation; dry mouth; lightheadedness; drowsiness; restlessness; tremors; *photosensitivity; menstrual changes; breast enlargement; impotence; retarded ejaculation; palpitations; *involuntary movements of face, jaw, tongue, and mouth; *blood, *liver, *heart, and *endocrine disorders; rash and other allergic reactions*

Dextroamphetamine sulfate [D] [I]
Brand: Dexedrine (Smith Kline & French)
Capsule, Tablet, Liquid
Indications: narcolepsy; attention deficit disorders, including childhood hyperactivity
Action: stimulates nervous system
Possible side effects: anorexia; nausea; diarrhea; abdominal cramps; nervousness; restlessness; dizziness; insomnia; headache; weight loss; reactive depression when discontinued; emotional disturbances; increased blood pressure; *rash and other allergic reactions*

Diazepam [D] [I]
Brand: Valium (Roche)
Tablet, Injection
Indications: anxiety; nervous tension; alcoholic withdrawal
Action: tranquilizes
Possible side effects: nausea; constipation; drowsiness; confusion; excitement; hallucinations; blurred vision; fluid retention; menstrual changes; *jaundice; rash and other allergic reactions*

Dihydroergocorine mesylate, dihydroergocristine mesylate, dihydroergocryptine mesylate [I]
Brand: Hydergine (Sandoz)
Tablet
Indications: depression; confusion and antisocial behavior in the elderly
Action: reduces depression, confusion, and antisocial behavior in the elderly
Possible side effects: nausea; dizziness; headache; *rash and other allergic reactions*

Drugs For The Mind

Type	Indications	Common Side Effects
major tranquilizers Thorazine Mellaril Stelazine Trilafon Haldol Navane	overwhelming anxiety paranoia hallucinations disorganized thinking	dry mouth; drowsiness; light-headedness; detached feeling; urinary difficulties; impotence; photosensitivity; tremor; inability to sit still; involuntary jerks or lip smacking
mild tranquilizers Librium Valium Serax Miltown Equanil	anxiety nervous tension	physical and psychological dependence; drowsiness; lightheadedness
anti-depressants Tofranil Elavil Sinequan Aventyl Parnate	unremitting depression with: suicidal ideas or intentions, early morning awakening, multiple bodily concerns, crying spells, agitation, hand-wringing, pacing, loss of libido, weight loss, constipation, insomnia	dry mouth; dizziness; drowsiness; impotence; urinary difficulties; constipation; irregular heartbeat
mood stabilizers lithium	mood swings, such as: intermittent depression ("lows") alternating with normal mood or elevated mood ("highs")	if dosage too high: tremors, confusion, coma, death
sleep medicines Dalmane Placidyl Doriden Seconal Nembutal	occasional insomnia	physical and psychological dependence; drowsiness; confusion
anti-sleep medicines nonprescription medicines	occasional need to stay awake	irritability, palpitations

Doxepin hydrochloride [I]
Brands: Sinequan (Pfizer), Adapin (Pennwalt)
Capsule, Liquid
Indication: depression
Action: relieves depression
Possible side effects: constipation; dry mouth; lightheadedness; drowsiness; blurred vision; dizziness; tremors;

impotence; *urinary difficulties; palpitations; hallucinations; *heart, *blood, and *liver disorders; rash and other allergic reactions

Ethchlorvynol D I
Brand: Placidyl (Abbott)
Capsule
Indication: occasional insomnia
Action: helps induce sleep
Possible side effects: nausea; vomiting; lightheadedness; confusion; blurred vision; dizziness; excitement; hangover; *liver and *blood disorders; rash and other allergic reactions

Flurazepam hydrochloride D I
Brand: Dalmane (Roche)
Capsule
Indication: occasional insomnia
Action: helps induce sleep
Possible side effects: nausea; constipation; drowsiness; confusion; excitement; hallucinations; blurred vision; fluid retention; menstrual changes; *jaundice; rash and other allergic reactions*

Glutethimide D I
Brand: Doriden (USV)
Tablet, Capsule
Indication: occasional insomnia
Action: helps induce sleep
Possible side effects: nausea; lightheadedness; confusion; excitement; blurred vision; hangover; *bone marrow depression; rash and other allergic reactions*

Haloperidol I
Brand: Haldol (McNeil)
Tablet, Liquid, Injection
Indications: anxiety; psychosis; Gilles de la Tourette's syndrome; hyperactive children
Action: tranquilizes
Possible side effects: constipation; dry mouth; lightheadedness; drowsiness; restlessness; tremors; *photosensitivity; menstrual changes; breast enlargement; impotence; retarded ejaculation; palpitations; *involuntary movements of face, jaw, tongue, and mouth; *blood, *liver, *heart, and *endocrine disorders; rash and other allergic reactions*

Hydroxyzine hydrochloride I
Brand: Atarax (Roerig)
Tablet, Liquid
Indications: anxiety; nervous tension; alcoholic withdrawal; nausea; vomiting; hives
Actions: tranquilizes; reduces congestion and inflammation (antihistamine)
Possible side effects: dry mouth; drowsiness; confusion; tremors; *rash and other allergic reactions*

Hydroxyzine pamoate I
Brand: Vistaril (Pfizer)
Capsule, Liquid
Indications: anxiety; nervous tension; itching
Action: tranquilizes
Possible side effects: dry mouth; drowsiness; confusion; *rash and other allergic reactions*

Imipramine hydrochloride I

Brand: Tofranil (Geigy)

Tablet

Indication: depression

Action: relieves depression

Possible side effects: constipation; dry mouth; lightheadedness; drowsiness; blurred vision; dizziness; tremors; impotence; *urinary difficulties; palpitations; hallucinations; *heart, *blood, and *liver disorders; rash and other allergic reactions*

Lithium carbonate [I]

Generic manufacturer: Philips Roxane

Brands: Eskalith (Smith Kline & French), Lithane (Dome), Lithobid, Lithonate, Lithotabs (Rowell)

Capsule, Tablet

Indications: mood swings; extreme high mood (mania)

Actions: reduces occurrence and severity of extreme high and low moods; reduces extreme high mood

Possible side effects: nausea; vomiting; diarrhea; drowsiness; diminished coordination; blurred vision; slurred speech; restlessness; fatigue; confusion; dizziness; headache; tremors; muscle spasms; fluid retention; urinary frequency; thyroid changes; *irregular heartbeat; rash and other allergic reactions*

Lorazepam [D] [I]

Brand: Ativan (Wyeth)

Tablet

Indications: anxiety; nervous tension; insomnia

Action: tranquilizes

Possible side effects: nausea; sedation; diminished coordination; confusion; dizziness; increased agitation; headache; weakness; increased perspiring; appetite changes

Meprobamate [D] [I]

Generic manufacturers: Premo, Purepac, Rexall

Brands: Equanil (Wyeth) Miltown, Miltown 600 (Wallace)

Tablet, Capsule

Indications: anxiety; nervous tension

Action: tranquilizes

Possible side effects: nausea; diarrhea; drowsiness; diminished coordination; blurred vision; slurred speech; dizziness; palpitations; *bone marrow depression; rash and other allergic reactions*

Methylphenidate hydrochloride [D] [I]

Brand: Ritalin (CIBA)

Tablet

Indications: narcolepsy; attention deficit disorders, including childhood hyperactivity

Action: stimulates nervous system

Possible side effects: anorexia; nausea; diarrhea; abdominal cramps; nervousness; restlessness; dizziness; insomnia; headache; weight loss; reactive depression when discontinued; emotional disturbances; increased blood pressure; *rash and other allergic reactions*

Nortriptyline hydrochloride [I]

Brand: Aventyl (Lilly)

Capsule, Liquid

Indication: depression

Action: relieves depression

Possible side effects: constipation; dry mouth; lightheadedness; drowsiness; blurred vision; dizziness; tremors; impotence; *urinary difficulties; palpitations; hallucinations; *heart, *blood, and *liver disorders; rash and other*

allergic reactions
Oxazepam   D   I
Brand: Serax (Wyeth)
Capsule, Tablet
Indications: anxiety; nervous tension; alcoholic withdrawal
Action: tranquilizes
Possible side effects: nausea; constipation; drowsiness; confusion; excitement; hallucinations; blurred vision; fluid retention; menstrual changes; *jaundice; rash and other allergic reactions*

Pentobarbital   D   I
Brand: Nembutal Elixer
Liquid
Indication: occasional insomnia
Action: helps induce sleep
Possible side effects: nausea; vomiting; drowsiness; lethargy; hangover; headache; *breathing difficulties; rash and other allergic reactions*

Perphenazine   I
Brand: Trilafon (Schering)
Tablet, Liquid, Injection
Indications: psychosis; anxiety; hyperactivity in children
Action: tranquilizes
Possible side effects: constipation; dry mouth; lightheadedness; drowsiness; restlessness; tremors; *photosensitivity; menstrual changes; breast enlargement; impotence; retarded ejaculation; palpitations; *involuntary movements of face, jaw, tongue, and mouth; *blood, *liver, *heart, and *endocrine disorders; rash and other allergic reactions*

Prochlorperazine. See *Gastrointestinal System*
Promethazine. See *Ear, Nose, and Throat*
Secobarbital   D   I
Brand: Seconal (Lilly)
Capsule, Liquid
Indication: occasional insomnia
Action: helps induce sleep
Possible side effects: nausea; vomiting; drowsiness; lethargy; hangover; headache; *breathing difficulties; rash and other allergic reactions*

Sodium butabarbital   D   I
Brands: Buticaps, Butisol Sodium (McNeil)
Tablet, Liquid, Capsule
Indication: occasional insomnia
Action: helps induce sleep
Possible side effects: nausea; vomiting; drowsiness; lethargy; hangover; headache; *breathing difficulties; rash and other allergic reactions*

Thioridazine hydrochloride   D   I
Brand: Mellaril (Sandoz)
Tablet, Liquid
Indications: psychosis; anxiety; hyperactivity in children
Action: tranquilizes
Possible side effects: constipation; dry mouth; lightheadedness; drowsiness; restlessness; tremors; *photosensitivity; menstrual changes; breast enlargement; impotence; retarded ejaculation; palpitations; *involuntary movements of face, jaw, tongue, and mouth; *blood, *liver, *heart, and *endocrine disorders; rash and other allergic reactions*

Thiothixene   I

Brand: Navane (Roerig)
Capsule, Liquid, Injection
Indications: anxiety; psychosis
Action: tranquilizes
Possible side effects: constipation; dry mouth; lightheadedness; drowsiness; restlessness; tremors; *photosensitivity; menstrual changes; breast enlargement; impotence; retarded ejaculation; palpitations; *involuntary movements of face, jaw, tongue, and mouth; *blood, *liver, *heart, and *endocrine disorders; rash and other allergic reactions*

Tranylcypromine sulfate D   I
Brand: Parnate (Smith Kline & French)
Tablet
Indication: depression
Action: relieves depression
Possible side effects: anorexia; nausea; diarrhea; constipation; dry mouth; restlessness; insomnia; blurred vision; dizziness; headache; weakness; muscle spasm; tremors; *palpitations; rash and other allergic reactions*
Note: avoid protein foods that are aged or have been flavor-enhanced by protein breakdown, such as cheese, sour cream, Chianti wine, sherry, beer, pickled herring, liver, canned figs, raisins, bananas or avocados, chocolate, soy sauce, broad bean pods, yeast extracts, or tenderized meat

Trifluoperazine hydrochloride I
Brand: Stelazine (Smith Kline & French)
Tablet
Indications: anxiety; psychosis
Action: tranquilizes
Possible side effects: constipation; dry mouth; lightheadedness; drowsiness; restlessness; tremors; *photosensitivity; menstrual changes; breast enlargement; impotence; retarded ejaculation; palpitations; *involuntary movements of face, jaw, tongue, and mouth; *blood, *liver, *heart, and *endocrine disorders; rash and other allergic reactions*

NONPRESCRIPTION DRUGS

Miles Nervine Nighttime Sleep-Aid (Miles)
Tablet
Indication: occasional insomnia
Action: sedates
No Doz (Bristol-Myers)
Tablet
Indication: drowsiness
Action: stimulates nervous system
Quiet World (Whitehall)
Tablet
Indication: occasional insomnia
Action: sedates
Sleep-Eze (Whitehall)
Tablet
Indication: insomnia
Action: sedates
Sominex (J.B. Williams)
Tablet
Indication: insomnia
Actions: sedates; reduces congestion and inflammation

(antihistamine)
Unisom (Leeming)
Tablet
Indication: insomnia
Actions: sedates; reduces congestion and inflammation (antihistamine)
Vivarin (J.B. Williams)
Tablet
Indication: drowsiness
Action: stimulates nervous system

Weight

Most weight reducing pills decrease appetite and stimulate the nervous system. This stimulation often causes irritability, nervousness, and insomnia. (Ironically, some people try to relieve these side effects by eating.) The drugs do not "burn up" fat; therefore, higher daily dosages will not cause rapid weight reduction. Continual use of appetite suppressants is not advised because the drugs lose their effectiveness and lead to abuse, dependence, and personality changes. Chronic obesity may be a sign of an underlying medical problem, particularly hormone problems such as diabetes or hypothyroidism; however, the most common cause of obesity is a combination of high-caloric diets and limited exercise. Medication alone will not alter these aspects of an individual's lifestyle. Adults must remember that their daily caloric requirements decrease about 15% every decade of life (excess calories are stored as fat). Finally, swelling of the legs or abdomen (edema) must be distinguished from obesity. If the swelling is caused by heart or kidney problems, diet pills may seriously aggravate these conditions.

PRESCRIPTION DRUGS
Diethylpropion hydrochloride [D] [I]
Brand: Tenuate (Merrell-National)
Tablet
Indication: obesity
Action: suppresses appetite
Possible side effects: nausea; vomiting; diarrhea; constipation; dry mouth; drowsiness; nervousness; restlessness; dizziness; insomnia; headache; tremors; impotence; increased blood pressure; personality change; palpitations; menstrual changes; *bone marrow depression; rash and other allergic reactions*
Phentermine hydrochloride [D] [I]
Brand: Fastin (Beecham)
Capsule
Indication: obesity
Action: suppresses appetite
Possible side effects: nausea; vomiting; diarrhea; constipation; dry mouth; drowsiness; nervousness; restlessness; dizziness; insomnia; headache; tremors; impotence; increased blood pressure; personality change; palpitations; menstrual changes; *bone marrow depression; rash and other allergic reactions*
Phentermine resin [D] [I]
Brand: Ionamin (Pennwalt)
Indication: obesity
Action: suppresses appetite
Possible side effects: nausea; vomiting; diarrhea; constipa-

tion; dry mouth; drowsiness; nervousness; restlessness; dizziness; insomnia; headache; tremors; impotence; increased blood pressure; personality change; palpitations; menstrual changes; *bone marrow depression; rash and other allergic reactions*

NONPRESCRIPTION DRUGS

Anorexin (SDA)
Capsule
Indication: obesity
Actions: suppresses appetite; stimulates nervous system

Appedrine, Extra Strength (Thompson)
Tablet
Indication: obesity
Actions: suppresses appetite; stimulates nervous system

Bio Slim T (Garden)
Capsule
Indication: obesity
Actions: suppresses appetite; stimulates nervous system

Dex-A-Diet II (O'Connor)
Capsule, Drops
Indication: obesity
Actions: suppresses appetite; stimulates nervous system

Dexatrim, Dexatrim Extra Strength (Thompson)
Capsule
Indication: obesity
Actions: suppresses appetite; stimulates nervous system

Diadax (O'Connor)
Capsule, Tablet
Indication: obesity
Actions: suppresses appetite; stimulates nervous system

Dietac (Menley & James)
Capsule, Tablet, Drops
Indication: obesity
Actions: suppresses appetite; stimulates nervous system

Fluidex (O'Connor)
Tablet
Indication: fluid retention
Action: reduces fluid retention

Fluidex-Plus (O'Connor)
Tablet
Indication: obesity
Actions: suppresses appetite; reduces fluid retention; stimulates nervous system

Hungrex Plus (Alleghany)
Tablet
Indication: obesity
Actions: suppresses appetite; reduces fluid retention; stimulates nervous system

Prolamine, Super Strength (Thompson)
Capsule
Indication: obesity
Actions: suppresses appetite; stimulates nervous system

P.V.M. (J.B. Williams)
Tablet
Indication: obesity
Actions: suppresses appetite; stimulates nervous system

Slim One Capsules (Garden)
Capsule
Indication: obesity
Action: suppresses appetite

Pain

Pain is the most common symptom of all illnesses. Drugs that treat the illness will therefore secondarily relieve the pain. Many of these drugs are not in themselves pain medications and are listed in the guide under the primary illness category. For example, drugs that relieve painful muscle spasms are listed in the section on the Musculo-Skeletal System.

Aspirin is the most commonly used medication for pain. This drug works both in the brain and at the affected area to relieve pain, and also reduces the inflammation and fever produced by the underlying problem. The main side effect of aspirin is gastric distress, which may be helped by taking the drug with milk. Acetaminophen (Tylenol) has the advantage of being less upsetting in the stomach, but some people find the drug is less helpful than aspirin in reducing inflammation. Most nonprescription pain medications contain either aspirin or acetaminophen; some are combined with buffers, bicarbonate, and caffeine as well as less powerful pain medicines. The advantage of these combinations over aspirin or acetaminophen alone is difficult to document.

The more potent pain medications require a doctor's prescription. Many of these drugs (Codeine, Darvon, Talwin, Demerol, etc.) are associated with the development of tolerance and physical dependency if used continuously for a period of time. Tolerance means that the body becomes affected by—"tolerant" to—a certain amount of the drug so that a larger dosage is required to provide the same degree of pain relief. The first sign of tolerance is that the usual dosage does not provide the same *duration* of pain relief; for example, whereas two pills used to provide relief for four hours, now the two pills only last three hours. To obtain the same degree of relief, one must then either take two pills more often or increase the dosage.

Physical dependency means that the body will have a physiological reaction if the pain medication is abruptly stopped; for example, one may have diarrhea, running nose, goose flesh, stomach cramps, and feel anxious or upset. Usually physical dependence upon a pain medication goes unnoticed because the pain does *not* stop suddenly but instead gradually subsides. The individual therefore takes less and less medicine over the period of a few days and "withdraws" from the higher dosage gradually without ever knowing that physical dependency has developed. If, however, the pain does stop all at once and symptoms of withdrawal do occur when the pain medicines are suddenly discontinued, the individual needs take only 1/4 the previous dosage to stop the reaction and then taper that amount over the next several days.

Tolerance and physical dependence are pharmacological effects of certain pain medications and should not be confused with psychological dependence or drug addiction. A person can become psychologically dependent on any drug and crave that drug and feel upset if that drug is withheld. Drug addiction is a complex pattern of drug-seeking behavior caused by psychological factors beyond the drug itself. Many addicts are *not* physically dependent on a drug.

The unrealistic fear of becoming psychologically or physically dependent on pain medication prevents some people from taking pain medication in the most effective way. Pain medicines work best *before* the pain becomes severe; they *prevent* pain from increasing far better than they reduce pain after it develops. For this reason, one should try to intercept the pain early and not try to endure the pain until it increases. Higher dosages may then be required to provide effective relief. When the pain is chronic and not related to an acute, time-limited illness, drugs alone may not be sufficient to provide relief and supplementary treatments may be necessary. such as hypnosis, self-relaxation, bio-feedback, or psychotherapy.

PRESCRIPTION DRUGS

Acetaminophen, chlorzoxazone. See *Musculo-Skeletal System*

Aspirin, caffeine, orphenadrine citrate, phenacetin. See *Musculo-Skeletal System*

Aspirin, phenacetin, caffeine, codeine phosphate [D] [I]
Brands: Empirin with Codeine, Empracet (Burroughs Wellcome)
Tablet
Indications: pain; fever; inflammation
Actions: relieves pain; reduces fever and inflammation
Possible side effects: nausea; vomiting; constipation; drowsiness; nervousness; flushing; lightheadedness; headache; *liver and *blood disorders; rash and other allergic reactions*

Brompheniramine maleate, guaifenesin, phenylephrine hydrochloride, phenylpropanolamine hydrochloride, codeine phosphate. See *Ear, Nose, and Throat*

Butalbital, aspirin, phenacetin, caffeine. See *Nervous System*

Carbamazepine. See *Nervous System*

Carisoprodol. See *Musculo-Skeletal System*

Codeine phosphate, acetaminophen [D] [I]
Brands: Phenaphen with Codeine (Robins), Tylenol with Codeine (McNeil)
Capsule, Tablet
Indications: pain; fever
Actions: relieves pain; reduces fever
Possible side effects: nausea; vomiting; constipation; drowsiness; lightheadedness; confusion; dizziness; hoarseness; *blood disorders*

Codeine sulfate, bromodiphenhydramine hydrochloride, diphenhydramine hydrochloride, ammonium chloride, potassium guaiacolsulfonate. See *Ear, Nose, and Throat*

Colchicine. See *Musculo-Skeletal System*

Dihydrocodeine, promethazine hydrochloride, aspirin, phenacetin, caffeine [D] [I]
Brand: Synalgos-DC (Ives)
Capsule
Indication: pain
Action: relieves pain
Possible side effects: nausea; vomiting; constipation; lightheadedness; sedation; dizziness; *rash and other allergic reactions*

Fenoprofen calcium. See *Musculo-Skeletal System*

Ibuprofen. See *Musculo-Skeletal System*

Indomethacin. See *Musculo-Skeletal System*

Levorphanol tartrate [D] [I]
Brand: Levo-Dromoran (Roche)
Tablet, Injection

Indication: pain

Action: relieves pain

Possible side effects: nausea; vomiting; dizziness; increased perspiring; respiratory depression; urinary retention; *rash and other allergic reactions*

Meperidine hydrochloride   ⬜D⬜   ⬜I⬜

Brand: Demerol (Winthrop)

Tablet, Liquid, Injection

Indication: pain

Actions: relieves pain; sedates

Possible side effects: nausea; vomiting; constipation; dry mouth; lightheadedness; sedation; restlessness; disorientation; diminished coordination; dizziness; flushing; increased perspiring; euphoria; weakness; vision disturbances; hallucinations; urinary retention; palpitations; irregular heartbeat; *rash and other allergic reactions*

Meprobamate, ethoheptazine citrate, aspirin. See *Nervous System*

Metaxalone. See *Musculo-Skeletal System*

Methadone hydrochloride   ⬜D⬜   ⬜I⬜

Brand: Dolophine Hydrochloride (Lilly)

Tablet, Injection

Indication: pain

Action: relieves pain

Possible side effects: nausea; vomiting; constipation; dry mouth; lightheadedness; sedation; restlessness; disorientation; diminished coordination; dizziness; flushing; increased perspiring; euphoria; weakness; vision disturbances; hallucinations; urinary retention; palpitations; irregular heartbeat; *rash and other allergic reactions*

Methenamine, phenyl salicylate, gelsemium, methylene blue, benzoic acid, atropine sulfate, hyoscyamine. See *Urogenital System*

Methocarbamol. See *Musculo-Skeletal System*

Methysergide maleate. See *Nervous System*

Naproxen. See *Musculo-Skeletal System*

Orphenadrine citrate. See *Musculo-Skeletal System*

Oxycodone hydrochloride, acetaminophen   ⬜D⬜   ⬜I⬜

Brand: Percocet-5 (Endo)

Tablet

Indications: pain; fever

Actions: relieves pain; reduces fever

Possible side effects: nausea; vomiting; constipation; drowsiness; sedation; lightheadedness; restlessness; euphoria; diminished coordination; dizziness; *rash and other allergic reactions*

Oxycodone hydrochloride, oxycodone terephthalate, aspirin, phenacetin, caffeine   ⬜D⬜   ⬜I⬜

Brand: Percodan (Endo)

Tablet

Indications: pain; fever; inflammation

Actions: relieves pain; reduces fever and inflammation

Possible side effects: constipation; gastrointestinal upset and bleeding; drowsiness; lightheadedness; diminished coordination; dizziness; ringing in ears; *rash and other allergic reactions*

Oxyphenbutazone. See *Musculo-Skeletal System*

Pentazocine hydrochloride   ⬜D⬜   ⬜I⬜

Brand: Talwin 50 (Winthrop)

Tablet

Indication: pain

Action: relieves pain

Possible side effects: anorexia; nausea; vomiting; diarrhea; constipation; drowsiness; lightheadedness; sedation; dizziness; vision disturbances; headache; emotional disturbances; urinary retention; palpitations; *rash and other allergic reactions*

Phenazopyridine hydrochloride. See *Urogenital System*

Phenobarbital, hyoscyamine sulfate, atropine sulfate, hyoscine hydrobromide. See *Gastrointestinal System*

Phenylbutazone. See *Musculo-Skeletal System*

Phenylbutazone, dried aluminum hydroxide gel, magnesium trisilicate. See *Musculo-Skeletal System*

Promethazine hydrochloride, potassium guaiacolsulfonate, codeine phosphate. See *Ear, Nose, and Throat*

Promethazine hydrochloride, potassium guaiacolsulfonate, phenylephrine hydrochloride, codeine phosphate. See *Ear, Nose, and Throat*

Propoxyphene hydrochloride 〔D〕 〔I〕

Brand: Darvon (Lilly)

Capsule

Indication: pain

Action: relieves pain

Possible side effects: nausea; vomiting; constipation; drowsiness; lightheadedness; excitability; insomnia; *rash and other allergic reactions*

Propoxyphene hydrochloride, aspirin, phenacetin, caffeine 〔D〕 〔I〕

Brand: Darvon Compound-65 (Lilly)

Capsule

Indications: pain; fever; inflammation

Actions: relieves pain; reduces fever and inflammation

Possible side effects: nausea; vomiting; abdominal cramps; constipation; drowsiness; lightheadedness; excitability; sedation; vision disturbances; insomnia; dizziness; headache; euphoria; weakness; **liver disorders; rash and other allergic reactions*

See also listing for Propoxyphene hydrochloride

Propoxyphene napsylate, acetaminophen 〔D〕 〔I〕

Brands: Darvocet-N 50, Darvocet-N 100 (Lilly)

Tablet

Indications: pain; fever

Actions: relieves pain; reduces fever

Possible side effects: nausea; vomiting; abdominal cramps; constipation; drowsiness; lightheadedness; excitability; sedation; vision disturbances; insomnia; dizziness; headache; euphoria; weakness; **liver disorders; rash and other allergic reactions*

Sulfisoxazole, phenazopyridine hydrochloride. See *Urogenital System*

Sulindac. See *Musculo-Skeletal System*

Tolmetin sodium. See *Musculo-Skeletal System*

Zomepirac sodium

Brand: Zomax (McNeil)

Tablet

Indications: pain, fever; inflammation

Actions: relieves pain; reduces fever and inflammation

Possible side effects: nausea; vomiting; abdominal cramps; diarrhea; constipation; drowsiness; nervousness; insomnia; dizziness; ringing in ears; increased perspiring; palpitations; *increased risk of intestinal bleeding or urinary tract infection; rash and other allergic reactions*

NONPRESCRIPTION DRUGS

Acephen Acetaminophen (G & W)
Suppository
Indications: pain; fever
Actions: relieves pain; reduces fever
Acetaminophen (Lederle)
Capsule, Tablet; Liquid
Indications: pain, fever
Actions: relieves pain; reduces fever
Alka Seltzer Effervescent Antacid & Analgesic. See *Gastro-intestinal System*
Anacin Analgesic (Whitehall)
Tablet
Indications: pain; fever; inflammation
Actions: relieves pain; reduces fever and inflammation
Anacin, Maximum Strength (Whitehall)
Tablet
Indications: pain; fever; inflammation
Actions: relieves pain; reduces fever and inflammation
Anacin-3 (Whitehall)
Tablet
Indications: pain; fever; inflammation
Actions: relieves pain; reduces fever and inflammation
Anuphen Suppositories (Comatic)
Suppository
Indications: pain; fever
Actions: relieves pain; reduces fever
Ascriptin. See *Musculo-Skeletal System*
Ascriptin A/D. See *Musculo-Skeletal System*
Aspercreme. See *Musculo-Skeletal System*
Aspirin Suppositories (Comatic)
Suppository
Indications: pain; fever; inflammation
Actions: relieves pain; reduces fever and inflammation
Bayer Aspirin, Bayer Children's Chewable Aspirin (Glen-brook)
Tablet
Indications: pain; fever; inflammation
Actions: relieves pain; reduces fever and inflammation
Bayer Timed-Release Aspirin (Glenbrook)
Tablet
Indications: pain; fever; cold; flu; headache; arthritis
Actions: relieves pain; reduces fever and inflammation
BiCozene Creme. See *Skin, Hair, and Scalp*
Bufferin (Bristol-Myers)
Tablet
Indications: pain; fever; cold; flu; headache; arthritis
Actions: relieves pain; reduces fever and inflammation
Calamatum. See *Skin, Hair, and Scalp*
Congespirin (Bristol-Myers)
Liquid
Indications: pain; fever
Actions: relieves pain; reduces fever
Datril (Bristol-Myers)
Tablet
Indications: pain; fever; sinus congestion; cold
Actions: relieves pain and congestion; reduces fever
Datril 500 (Bristol-Myers)
Tablet
Indications: pain; headache; fever

Actions: relieves pain; reduces fever

Dibucaine Ointment. See *Skin, Hair, and Scalp*

Empirin (Burroughs Wellcome)

Tablet

Indications: pain; fever

Actions: relieves pain; reduces fever

Excedrin (Bristol-Myers)

Tablet

Indications: headache; pain; sinus pain; cold; flu; muscle ache; arthritis

Actions: relieves pain; reduces fever and inflammation

Liquiprin (Norcliff Thayer)

Liquid

Indications: pain; fever; cold; flu

Actions: relieves pain; reduces fever

Midol. See *Urogenital System*

Oraphen-PD (Comatic)

Liquid

Indications: pain; headache; fever

Actions: relieves pain; reduces fever

Ornex (Menley & James)

Capsule

Indications: pain; cold; flu; sinus congestion

Actions: relieves pain and congestion; reduces fever

Panalgesic (Poythress)

Liquid

Indications: pain; muscle ache

Action: relieves pain

Percogesic Tablets (Endo)

Tablet

Indications: pain; headache; muscle and joint soreness; neuralgia; sinusitis; menstrual cramps; cold; toothache; rheumatism; arthritis

Action: relieves pain

St. Joseph Aspirin for Children (Plough)

Tablet

Indications: pain; fever; inflammation

Actions: relieves pain; reduces fever and inflammation

Solarcaine. See *Skin, Hair, and Scalp*

Tempra (Mead Johnson)

Liquid

Indications: pain; fever

Actions: relieves pain; reduces fever

Tylenol (McNeil)

Tablet

Indications: pain; fever

Actions: relieves pain; reduces fever

Tylenol Children's Chewable Tablets, Elixir, Drops (McNeil)

Tablet, Liquid

Indications: pain; fever

Actions: relieves pain; reduces fever

Tylenol Extra-Strength (McNeil)

Capsule, Tablet, Liquid

Indications: pain; fever

Actions: relieves pain; reduces fever

Viro-Med (Whitehall)

Liquid, Tablet

Indications: pain; cold; flu

Actions: relieves pain and cough; reduces fever; loosens phlegm

Respiratory System

Medicines that are intended for the relief of a cough can act to suppress the cough reflex, to loosen phlegm so it can be coughed up, or to dry up the phlegm. Because the drugs have different actions, the time of day determines which drug would be most helpful. For example, at bedtime a cough suppressant will aid peaceful sleep, while a drug to loosen phlegm so that it can be coughed up is preferable during the day. When a drug has a combination of ingredients, they sometimes work against one another, such as simultaneously loosening phlegm and suppressing cough.

For chronic lung diseases (such as asthma, emphysema, and bronchitis), the patient must establish a trusting and sustained relationship with a doctor because many drugs will have to be tried and adjusted over time. The kind of drug along with the dosage and frequency will depend on the individual, the season, the emotional situation, and the state of the disease.

PRESCRIPTION DRUGS

Aminophylline A E
Brand: Aminophyllin (Searle)
Tablet
Indications: asthma; bronchitis; emphysema
Actions: dilates bronchial tubes; reduces fluid retention; stimulates cardiac muscles
Possible side effects: anorexia; nausea; vomiting; lightheadedness; nervousness; dizziness; flushing; headache; palpitations; *rash and other allergic reactions*

Beclomethasone dipropionate
Brand: Vanceril (Schering)
Aerosol inhaler
Indication: asthma
Action: reduces inflammation
Possible side effects: dry mouth; hoarseness; *throat fungal infections; rash and other allergic reactions*
Warning: transference from systemic corticosteroid treatment to Beclomethasone treatment can make adrenal insufficiency apparent

Betamethasone. See *Cancer*

Brompheniramine maleate. See *Allergies*

Brompheniramine maleate, guaifenesin, phenylephrine hydrochloride, phenylpropanolamine hydrochloride. See *Ear, Nose, and Throat*

Brompheniramine maleate, guaifenesin, phenylephrine hydrochloride, phenylpropanolamine hydrochloride, codeine phosphate. See *Ear, Nose, and Throat*

Brompheniramine maleate, phenylephrine hydrochloride, phenylpropanolamine hydrochloride. See *Ear, Nose, and Throat*

Caramiphen edisylate, chlorpheniramine maleate, phenylpropanolamine hydrochloride, isopropamide iodide D
Brand: Tuss-Ornade (Smith Kline & French)
Capsule, Liquid
Indications: cough; congestion
Actions: suppresses cough; reduces congestion
Possible side effects: anorexia; nausea; vomiting; diarrhea; constipation; abdominal cramps; dry mouth; drowsiness; dizziness; nervousness; headache; palpitations; blurred

vision; *urinary difficulties; *rash and other allergic reactions*

Cephalexin. See *Infection*

Chlorpheniramine maleate. See *Allergies*

Chlorpheniramine maleate, phenylpropanolamine hydrochloride, isopropamide iodide. See *Ear, Nose, and Throat*

Codeine phosphate, guaifenesin, pseudoephedrine hydrochloride, triprolidine hydrochloride ⬚D ⬚I

Brand: Actifed-C Expectorant (Burroughs Wellcome)

Liquid

Indications: cough; congestion; pain

Actions: suppresses cough; reduces congestion

Possible side effects: anorexia; nausea; vomiting; diarrhea; constipation; abdominal cramps; dry mouth; drowsiness; dizziness; nervousness; headache; palpitations; blurred vision; *urinary difficulties; *rash and other allergic reactions*

Codeine sulfate, bromodiphenhydramine hydrochloride, diphenhydramine hydrochloride, ammonium chloride, potassium guaiacolsulfonate. See *Ear, Nose, and Throat*

Dexbrompheniramine maleate, pseudoephedrine sulfate. See *Ear, Nose, and Throat*

Dexchlorpheniramine maleate. See *Allergies*

Ephedrine sulfate, theophylline, hydroxyzine hydrochloride ⬚I

Brand: Marax (Roerig)

Tablet, Liquid

Indication: asthma

Action: relaxes bronchial muscles

Possible side effects: nausea; vomiting; dizziness; nervousness; insomnia; headache; increased perspiring; palpitations; *urinary difficulties

See also listing for Theophylline

Epinephrine hydrochloride. See *Allergies*

Erythromycin. See *Infection*

Isoproterenol hydrochloride

Brand: Aerolone (Lilly)

Liquid spray

Indications: asthma; bronchitis; emphysema

Action: relaxes bronchial muscles

Possible side effects: nausea; vomiting; dizziness; nervousness; insomnia; headache; weakness; palpitations; *urinary difficulties

Metaproterenol sulfate

Brand: Alupent (Boehringer Ingelheim)

Tablet, Liquid, Spray

Indications: asthma; bronchitis; emphysema

Action: relaxes bronchial muscles

Possible side effects: nausea; vomiting; dizziness; nervousness; insomnia; headache; weakness; palpitations; *urinary difficulties

Oxtriphylline

Brand: Choledyl (Parke-Davis)

Tablet, Liquid

Indication: asthma

Action: dilates bronchial tubes

Possible side effects: nausea; vomiting; nervousness; palpitations; *rash and other allergic reactions*

Penicillin V potassium. See *Infection*

Phenylpropanolamine hydrochloride, phenylephrine hydro-

Shortness Of Breath

Diagnosis	Physical Effects	Possible Treatments	Comments
cold or flu	congestion of larger airways	decongestants rest, fluids, aspirin cough suppressants antibiotics for secondary bacterial infection	recurrent or prolonged bouts require medical evaluation
asthma	inflammation and narrowing of smaller airways	avoidance of cause of allergy inhalants to relieve spasmodic constriction and congestion steroids to reduce allergic response and inflammation	indiscriminate overuse of medication can harmfully affect heart and blood pressure
chronic bronchitis	inflammation of large and small airways	avoidance of irritants, including tobacco smoke decongestants	treatment should begin before irreversible scarring occurs
emphysema	decreased elasticity of air pockets	avoidance of irritants, including tobacco smoke medication promptly if secondary infections occur	the best treatment is prevention of contributing causes
pneumonia	infection throughout one section of lungs	antibiotics for bacterial infections rest, fluids, aspirin decongestants	the disease stresses the entire body system in elderly or debilitated patients
tuberculosis	scarring and cavities in sections of lungs	antitubercular medication optimum nutrition and general health care	medication is still required long after disappearance of the symptoms
lung cancer	obstruction of airways and air pockets by tumor growth	cancer drugs radiation to diminish growth surgical removal of tumor	the prognosis improves with early detection
congestive heart failure	accumulation of fluid in lungs with decreased oxygen in blood	diuretics to remove excess fluid digitalis to strengthen heart contraction adjustment of heart rhythm reduction of high blood pressure	the early signs are shortness of breath when lying flat or walking up stairs
any serious illness (e.g. anemia, infection)	increased demand on lungs for oxygen	treatment of primary illness rest	shortness of breath can occur with illnesses unrelated to the respiratory system

chloride, **phenyltoloxamine citrate, chlorpheniramine maleate.** See *Ear, Nose, and Throat*

Prednisone oral. See *Musculo-Skeletal System*

Promethazine hydrochloride, potassium guaiacolsulfonate. See *Ear, Nose, and Throat*

Promethazine hydrochloride, potassium guaiacolsulfonate, codeine phosphate. See *Ear, Nose, and Throat*

Promethazine hydrochloride, potassium guaiacolsulfonate, phenylephrine hydrochloride. See *Ear, Nose, and Throat*

Promethazine hydrochloride, potassium guaiacolsulfonate, phenylephrine hydrochloride, codeine phosphate. See *Ear, Nose, and Throat*

Pseudoephedrine hydrochloride, triprolidine hydrochloride. See *Ear, Nose, and Throat*

Terbutaline sulfate
Brand: Brethine (Geigy)
Tablet
Indication: asthma
Action: dilates bronchial tubes
Possible side effects: diarrhea; dizziness; anxiety; tremors; palpitations: *rash and other allergic reactions*

Tetracycline hydrochloride. See *Infection*

Theophylline [A] [E]
Brand: Elixophyllin (Berlex)
Capsule, Liquid
Indications: asthma; bronchitis; emphysema
Action: dilates bronchial tubes
Possible side effects: nausea; vomiting; diarrhea; abdominal cramps; restlessness; irritability; insomnia; headache; flushing; palpitations; *convulsions*

Theophylline, ephedrine hydrochloride, butabarbital
[A] [D] [E] [I]
Brand: Tedral-25 (Parke-Davis)
Tablet
Indication: bronchial spasm
Actions: dilates bronchial tubes; sedates
Possible side effects: nausea; vomiting; abdominal cramps; drowsiness; dizziness; agitation; tremors; headache; cold hands and feet; weakness; palpitations; *rash and other allergic reactions*
See also listing for Theophylline

Theophylline, ephedrine hydrochloride, phenobarbital
[A] [D] [E] [I]
Brands: Tedral, Tedral SA (Parke-Davis)
Tablet, Liquid
Indication: bronchial spasm
Actions: dilates bronchial tubes; sedates
Possible side effects: nausea; vomiting; abdominal cramps; drowsiness; dizziness; agitation; tremors; headache; cold hands and feet; weakness; palpitations; *rash and other allergic reactions*
See also listing for Theophylline

Theophylline, ephedrine hydrochloride, phenobarbital, guaifenesin [A] [D] [E] [I]
Brand: Tedral Expectorant (Parke-Davis)
Tablet
Indication: bronchial spasm and congestion
Actions: dilates bronchial tubes; sedates; loosens phlegm
Possible side effects: nausea; vomiting; abdominal cramps; drowsiness; dizziness; agitation; tremors; headache; cold hands and feet; weakness; palpitations; *rash and other*

allergic reactions
See also listing for Theophylline

Theophylline, guaifenesin A   E
Brand: Quibron (Mead Johnson)
Capsule, Liquid
Indications: asthma; congestion
Actions: relaxes bronchial muscles; reduces congestion
Possible side effects: nausea; vomiting; abdominal cramps;
   drowsiness; dizziness; agitation; tremors; headache; cold
   hands and feet; weakness; palpitations; *rash and other
   allergic reactions*
See also listing for Theophylline

Triamcinolone. See *Musculo-Skeletal System*

Tripelennamine hydrochloride, ephedrine sulfate. See *Allergies*

NONPRESCRIPTION DRUGS

Alka-Seltzer Plus (Miles)
Tablet
Indications: flu; cold; hay fever; nasal and sinus congestion
Action: reduces pain and congestion

Allerest. See *Allergies*

A.R.M. Allergy Relief Medicine. See *Allergies*

Bayer Children's Cold Tablets (Glenbrook)
Tablet
Indications: flu; cold; fever; sinus congestion
Actions: reduces fever; relieves pain and congestion

Bayer Cough Syrup for Children (Glenbrook)
Liquid
Indications: cough; sinus congestion
Actions: suppresses cough; relieves congestion

Bronkaid Mist (Winthrop)
Liquid spray
Indication: asthma
Action: reduces bronchial muscle spasm

Bronkaid Tablets (Winthrop)
Tablet
Indication: asthma
Actions: reduces bronchial spasm; loosens phlegm

Cheracol D Cough Syrup (Upjohn)
Liquid
Indication: cough
Action: relieves cough

Chloraseptic DM Cough Control. See *Ear, Nose, and Throat*

Chlor-Trimeton Allergy Syrup and Tablets. See *Allergies*

Chlor-Trimeton Decongestant (Schering)
Tablet
Indications: cold; flu; hay fever
Action: relieves congestion and sneezing

Chlor-Trimeton Expectorant. See *Ear, Nose, and Throat*

Comtrex (Bristol-Myers)
Tablet
Indications: cough; nasal congestion; cold; flu; fever; head-
   ache
Action: relieves cough and congestion

Congespirin. See *Pain*

Contac (Menley & James)
Capsule
Indication: congestion
Action: relieves congestion

Coricidin, Coricidin 'D' (Schering)

Tablet, Liquid, Spray

Indications: cough; congestion; pain

Actions: relieves pain and congestion; suppresses cough; reduces fever

Coricidin Medilets, Coricidin Demilets, Coricidin Cough Syrup (for children) (Schering)

Tablet, Liquid

Indications: cough; pain; fever

Actions: relieves pain, congestion, and cough; reduces fever

Coricidin Sinus Headache Tablets (Extra Strength). See *Ear, Nose, and Throat*

Coryban-D (Pfipharmecs)

Capsule

Indication: sinus congestion

Action: relieves congestion

Coryban-D Cough Syrup (Pfipharmecs)

Liquid

Indication: cough

Action: relieves cough

CoTylenol Cold Formula (McNeil)

Tablet

Indications: nasal congestion; fever; pain

Actions: reduces fever and pain; relieves congestion

CoTylenol Liquid Cold Formula (McNeil)

Liquid

Indications: cough; nasal congestion; fever; pain

Actions: relieves congestion and cough; reduces fever and pain

C3 (Menley & James)

Capsule

Indications: cough; congestion

Action: relieves cough and congestion

Datril. See *Pain*

Dristan-AF Decongestant (Whitehall)

Tablet

Indications: nasal congestion; fever; pain; hay fever

Actions: relieves congestion and pain; reduces fever

Dristan Decongestant (Whitehall)

Tablet, Capsule

Indications: nasal congestion; pain; fever; hay fever

Actions: relieves pain and congestion; reduces fever

Dristan Nasal Mist (Whitehall)

Mist (regular and menthol)

Indications: nasal congestion; cold; respiratory allergy

Action: relieves congestion

Fedahist Expectorant, Syrup, and Tablets (Dooner)

Liquid, Tablet

Indications: nasal inflammation; congestion

Actions: reduces congestion and inflammation (antihistamine); loosens phlegm

Formula 44 Cough Mixture (Vicks)

Liquid

Indications: cough; bronchitis; flu

Action: relieves cough

Formula 44D Decongestant Cough Mixture (Vicks)

Liquid

Indications: cough; congestion; flu

Actions: relieves congestion and cough; loosens phlegm and mucus

4-Way Cold Tablets (Bristol-Myers)

Tablet

Indications: pain; fever; nasal congestion; cold; respiratory allergy

Actions: relieves pain and congestion; reduces fever

4-Way Long Acting Mentholated Nasal Spray, 4-Way Long Acting Nasal Spray (Bristol-Myers)

Spray

Indications: nasal and sinus congestion; hay fever; respiratory allergy

Action: relieves congestion

Neo-Synephrine Hydrochloride (Winthrop)

Spray, Liquid (topical), Jelly

Indications: respiratory allergies; nasal and sinus congestion; hay fever

Action: relieves congestion

Neo-Synephrine II Long Acting (Winthrop)

Liquid (topical), Spray

Indications: respiratory allergies; nasal and sinus congestion; hay fever

Action: relieves congestion

Novahistine. See *Allergies*

Novahistine Cough Formula (Dow)

Liquid

Indication: cough

Action: relieves cough

Novahistine DMX (Dow)

Liquid

Indications: cough; nasal and sinus congestion

Action: relieves cough and congestion

Nyquil Nighttime Colds Medicine (Vicks)

Liquid

Indications: cough; nasal congestion; pain

Action: relieves pain, cough, and congestion

Ornex Capsules. See *Pain*

Primatene Mist (Whitehall)

Spray

Indication: asthma

Action: dilates bronchial tubes

Primatene Mist Suspension (Whitehall)

Aerosol spray

Indication: asthma

Action: dilates bronchial tubes

Primatene Tablets (Whitehall)

Tablet

Indications: asthma; hay fever

Action: dilates bronchial tubes

Rhinosyn-DM (Additive Free) (Comatic)

Liquid

Indications: cough; nasal and sinus congestion

Actions: relieves congestion; suppresses cough

Rhinosyn Syrup, Rhinosyn-PD. See *Ear, Nose, and Throat*

Rhinosyn-X (Additive Free) (Comatic)

Liquid

Indications: cough; nasal and sinus congestion

Action: loosens phlegm and bronchial secretions

Robitussin, Robitussin-DM (Robins)

Liquid

Indication: cough

Actions: loosens phlegm; relieves cough

Robitussin-CF (Robins)

Liquid
Indication: cough
Actions: relieves cough and congestion; loosens phlegm
Robitussin-PE (Robins)
Liquid
Indication: cough
Actions: relieves congestion; loosens phlegm
St. Joseph Cold Tablets for Children (Plough)
Tablet
Indications: nasal congestion; fever; pain
Actions: relieves congestion and pain; reduces fever
St. Joseph Cough Syrup for Children (Plough)
Liquid
Indication: cough during cold and flu
Action: suppresses cough
Sinarest Tablets. See *Allergies*
Sine-Off AF Aspirin-Free Extra Strength Tablets. See *Allergies*
Sine-Off Once-A-Day Sinus Spray (Menley & James)
Spray
Indication: nasal and sinus congestion
Action: relieves nasal and sinus congestion
Sine-Off Tablets-Aspirin Formula. See *Allergies*
Sinutab Extra Strength. See *Allergies*
Sinutab Long Lasting Decongestant Sinus Spray (Warner-Lambert)
Spray
Indication: nasal congestion
Action: relieves nasal congestion
Sinutab Tablets. See *Ear, Nose, and Throat*
Sinutab-II Tablets. See *Ear, Nose, and Throat*
Sucrets Cold Decongestant Formula. See *Ear, Nose, and Throat*
Sucrets Cough Control Formula. See *Ear, Nose, and Throat*
Symptom 1 (Parke-Davis)
Liquid
Indication: cough during cold
Action: suppresses cough
Symptom 2 (Parke-Davis)
Liquid
Indications: cough; nasal congestion
Action: relieves cough and nasal congestion
Triaminic-DM Cough Formula (Dorsey)
Liquid
Indications: cough; nasal congestion
Action: relieves cough and nasal congestion
Triaminic Expectorant (Dorsey)
Liquid
Indications: cough; nasal congestion
Action: relieves cough and nasal congestion
Triaminic Syrup. See *Allergies*
Triaminicin Tablets. See *Allergies*
Triaminicol Decongestant Cough Syrup (Dorsey)
Liquid
Indications: cough and congestion during cold
Actions: suppresses cough; reduces congestion
Vicks Cough Silencers Cough Drops. See *Ear, Nose, and Throat*
Vicks Cough Syrup (Vicks)
Liquid

Indications: cold; flu; bronchitis
Actions: relieves cough; loosens phlegm; soothes irritated throat
Vicks Sinex Long-Lasting Decongestant Nasal Spray. See *Allergies*
Viro-Med. See *Pain*

Skin, Hair, and Scalp

Skin is not simply a covering for the body. It is a complicated organ system that helps regulate body temperature, salts, and metabolism. Because every inch of this organ has many different microscopic parts, many different kinds of problems can arise. Therefore, an ointment stored in the medicine chest for one kind of skin problem in the past should not be used for a current skin problem even in the same area without the advice of a doctor. For example, if the lotion used in the past was for an *allergy*, it may make a current *infection* more widespread.

The skin has an elaborate system to protect the body against unwanted "foreign" substances. This protective system causes the skin to be quite sensitive to drugs. For this reason, the skin commonly is the first organ to reveal by a rash or itching a potential allergy. This warning signal of the skin should not be ignored and may forecast a more serious reaction of another part of the body. Also, because of this sensitivity of the skin, no drug or cosmetic agent should be applied widely until tested in a small area.

PRESCRIPTION DRUGS

Betamethasone valerate
Brand: Valisone (Schering)
Cream
Indication: skin inflammation
Action: reduces inflammation
Possible side effects: dryness; skin discoloration; hair follicle inflammation; *secondary infection; rash and other allergic reactions*
Cephalexin. See *Infection*
Clotrimazole
Brand: Lotrimin (Schering)
Cream, Liquid (topical)
Indication: fungal skin infections
Action: reduces fungus
Possible side effects: redness; stinging; irritation; swelling; blistering; peeling
Clotrimazole. See *Urogenital System*
Dexchlorpheniramine maleate. See *Allergies*
Diiodohydroxyquin, hydrocortisone. See *Infection*
Doxycycline. See *Infection*
Erythromycin. See *Infection*
Fluocinolone acetonide
Brand: Synalar (Syntex)
Cream, Ointment, Liquid (topical)
Indication: skin inflammation
Action: reduces inflammation
Possible side effects: dryness; skin discoloration; hair follicle inflammation; *secondary infection; rash and other allergic reactions*

Fluocinonide

Brands: Lidex (Syntex), Topsyn (Syntex)

Cream, Ointment, Gel

Indication: skin inflammation

Action: reduces inflammation

Possible side effects: dryness; skin discoloration; hair follicle inflammation; *secondary infection; rash and other allergic reactions*

Flurandrenolide

Brand: Cordran (Dista)

Cream, Ointment, Lotion

Indication: skin inflammation

Actions: reduces inflammation; narrows swollen blood vessels

Possible side effects: dryness; burning; *secondary infection; rash and other allergic reactions*

Gentamicin sulfate. See *Infection*

Hydroxyzine pamoate. See *Nervous System*

Iodochlorhydroxyquin, hydrocortisone

Brand: Vioform-Hydrocortisone (Ciba)

Ointment, Cream

Indication: skin inflammation and infection

Action: reduces fungus, bacteria, and inflammation

Possible side effects: dryness; itching; skin discoloration; hair follicle inflammation; burning; *secondary infection; rash and other allergic reactions*

Lindane (gamma benzene hexachloride)

Brand: Kwell (Reed & Carnrick)

Cream, Lotion, Shampoo

Indications: scabies; head lice; crab lice

Action: kills scabies and lice

Possible side effects: itching; *central nervous system toxicity, especially in children; rash and other allergic reactions*

Nystatin. See *Infection*

Nystatin, neomycin sulfate, gramicidin, triamcinolone acetonide

Brand: Mycolog (Squibb)

Cream, Ointment

Indication: skin inflammation and infection

Actions: reduces inflammation; treats infection

Possible side effects: dryness; itching; skin discoloration; hair follicle inflammation; burning; *secondary infection; rash and other allergic reactions*

See also listing for Triamcinolone acetonide

Sulfamethoxazole. See *Infection*

Tetracycline hydrochloride. See *Infection*

Triamcinolone acetonide

Brand: Kenalog (Squibb)

Cream, Lotion, Ointment, Spray

Indication: skin inflammation

Action: reduces inflammation

Possible side effects: dryness; itching; skin discoloration; hair follicle inflammation; burning; *secondary infection; rash and other allergic reactions*

Tripelennamine hydrochloride, ephedrine sulfate. See *Allergies*

NONPRESCRIPTION DRUGS

A and D Ointment (Schering)

Ointment

Indications: rash; cuts; burns

Actions: soothes; protects from wetness; lubricates
Aftate. See *Infection*
Alpha Keri (Westwood)
Liquid (topical), Soap
Indications: dry skin; itching
Action: moisturizes
Bactine. See *Infection*
Betadine. See *Infection*
BiCozene Creme (Creighton)
Cream
Indications: minor burns; sunburn; cuts; insect bites; abrasions; skin irritations; itching
Action: relieves pain and itching
Calamatum (Blair)
Liquid (topical), Spray, Ointment
Indications: skin irritations; poison ivy, oak, and sumac; insect bites; rashes; chafing
Actions: relieves pain and itching; soothes
Caldesene Medicated (Pharmacraft)
Powder, Ointment
Indication: rash
Actions: reduces bacteria; repels moisture
Clearasil (Vicks)
Cream, Lotion
Indication: acne
Actions: dries pimples; reduces bacteria
Compound W (Whitehall)
Liquid (topical)
Indication: warts
Action: aids in removal of warts
Cruex. See *Infection*
Denorex Medicated Shampoo (Whitehall)
Shampoo
Indications: dandruff; seborrhea; psoriasis
Action: reduces itching and flaking
Derma Medicone. See *Mouth and Teeth*
Desitin Ointment (Leeming)
Ointment
Indication: rash
Action: protects from wetness
Dibucaine Ointment (Comatic)
Ointment
Indication: painful skin conditions
Action: relieves pain
Eclipse: Original, Partial, Total (Herbert)
Lotion, Gel
Indications: sun exposure; skin cancer susceptibility; aging
Action: reduces sunburn
Eclipse After Sun Lotion (Herbert)
Lotion
Indication: dry skin
Action: moisturizes
Eclipse Sunscreen Lip and Face Protectant (Herbert)
Balm
Indications: sun and wind exposure; burning; chapping
Action: protects against dryness
Fostex BPO 5% (Westwood)
Gel
Indication: acne
Actions: reduces bacteria; dries oily skin
Fostex Cake (Westwood)

Soap
Indication: acne
Actions: reduces bacteria; dries oily skin
Fostex CM (Westwood)
Cream
Indication: acne
Actions: conceals blemishes; dries oily skin
Fostex Cream & Medicated Cleanser (Westwood)
Cream, Liquid (topical)
Indications: acne; dandruff
Actions: reduces bacteria; dries oily hair and skin
Freezone Solution (Whitehall)
Liquid (topical)
Indications: calluses; corns
Action: aids in removal of corns and calluses
Head and Shoulders (Procter & Gamble)
Shampoo (Lotion, Cream)
Indications: dandruff; seborrhea
Action: decreases itching and scaling
Keri Creme (Westwood)
Cream
Indication: dry skin
Action: moisturizes
Lanacane Medicated Creme. See *Urogenital System*
Listerine Antiseptic. See *Mouth and Teeth*
Mercurochrome. See *Infection*
Nupercainal. See *Pain*
Outgro (Whitehall)
Liquid
Indication: ingrown toenail
Actions: reduces swelling, inflammation, and pain; toughens skin
Pernox, Pernox Lotion (Westwood)
Ointment, Lotion, Shampoo
Indications: acne; oily skin and scalp
Action: dries oily skin and scalp
pHisoDerm (Winthrop)
Liquid (topical)
Indication: cleaning of skin, scalp, and hair
Actions: cleans skin, scalp, and hair; reduces bacteria
PreSun 4 Sunscreen Lotion, PreSun 15 Sunscreen Lotion, PreSun 8 (Westwood)
Lotion, Gel
Indications: sun exposure; skin cancer susceptibility; aging
Action: reduces sunburn
PreSun Sunscreen Lip Protection (Westwood)
Ointment
Indication: sun and wind exposure
Action: protects lips from drying and chapping
Rhulicaine (Lederle)
Aerosol
Indications: sunburn; minor skin irritations
Action: relieves pain
Rhulicream, Rhuligel, Rhulihist, Rhulispray (Lederle)
Ointment, Gel, Liquid (topical), Spray
Indications: poison ivy or oak; insect bites; skin irritations; sunburn
Action: relieves itching and pain
Rid (Pfipharmecs)
Liquid (topical)
Indication: head, body, or pubic lice

Actions: kills and aids removal of lice and eggs

Sebucare (Westwood)

Shampoo

Indications: dandruff; seborrhea; scaling

Action: decreases scaling, oil, and itching

Selsun Blue Lotion (Abbott)

Shampoo

Indication: dandruff

Action: decreases dandruff

Shade Sunscreen Lotion (SPF-6), Shade Plus Sunscreen Lotion (SPF-8) (Plough)

Lotion

Indications: sun exposure; skin cancer susceptibility; aging

Action: reduces sunburn

Solarcaine (Plough)

Cream, Spray (topical)

Indications: sunburn; minor burns; scrapes; cuts; chapping; poison ivy; insect bites

Action: reduces pain, itching, and inflammation

Sunbrella Sunscreen Lotion (5% PABA) (Dorsey)

Lotion

Indications: sun exposure; skin cancer susceptibility; aging

Action: reduces sunburn

Super Shade (SPF-15) (Plough)

Lotion

Indications: sun exposure; skin cancer susceptibility; aging

Action: reduces sunburn

Tegrin (Block)

Lotion, Cream

Indication: psoriasis

Action: controls itching and scaling

Tinactin. See *Infection*

Topex Acne Clearing Medication (Vicks)

Lotion

Indication: acne

Actions: dries; reduces bacteria

Unguentine Plus (Norwich-Eaton)

Cream

Indications: cuts; burns

Actions: cleans; relieves pain; moisturizes

Vanoxide Acne Lotion (Dermik)

Lotion

Indications: acne; oily skin

Actions: reduces bacteria; dries oily skin

Vergo (Daywell)

Ointment

Indication: warts

Action: aids in removal of warts

Wart-Off (Pfipharmecs)

Liquid (topical)

Indication: warts

Action: aids in removal of warts

Xylocaine 2.5% Ointment (Astra)

Ointment

Indications: burns; sunburn; irritations; hemorrhoids; insect bites

Action: reduces burning, itching, and pain

Zincon Dandruff Shampoo (Lederle)

Shampoo

Indication: dandruff

Action: decreases dandruff

Urogenital System

Symptoms of the lower portion of the urinary system include burning and frequent urination and a feeling of urgency despite limited amounts of urine. These symptoms commonly occur with infections that antibiotics can relieve. However, the individual should not treat recurrent infections without a determination of the underlying cause. In addition, the drug should be taken for the entire prescribed period. Even though the symptoms may disappear after only one or two days, the source of the infection may not have been adequately treated. An acute and minor problem can change to a severe, chronic one.

Symptoms of the upper portion of the urinary system, including the kidneys, often do not appear until the underlying disease is more advanced. For this reason a urine analysis is part of a routine examination to check on possible "silent" problems. If the doctor prescribes a drug for such an asymptomatic illness, such as a chronic kidney infection, the medicine should be taken diligently despite the lack of any apparent difficulty.

PRESCRIPTION DRUGS

Carbenicillin. See *Infection*

Cephalexin. See *Infection*

Chlorothiazide. See *Cardiovascular System*

Chlorthalidone. See *Cardiovascular System*

Clotrimazole
Brand: Gyne-Lotrimin (Schering)
Cream, Tablet
Indication: fungal infection of vaginal tract and skin
Action: reduces fungus
Possible side effects: irritation; itching; burning; urinary frequency; irritation of genitals of sexual partner

Cycloserine. See *Infection*

Doxycycline. See *Infection*

Erythromycin. See *Infection*

Furosemide. See *Cardiovascular System*

Hydrochlorothiazide. See *Cardiovascular System*

Hydrocortisone acetate, bismuth subgallate, bismuth resorcin, benzyl benzoate, Peruvian balsam, zinc oxide. See *Gastrointestinal System*

Methenamine, phenyl salicylate, gelsemium, methylene blue, benzoic acid, atropine sulfate, hyoscyamine
Brand: Trac Tabs (Hyrex)
Tablet
Indication: urinary tract infections
Actions: reduces bacteria; relieves pain
Possible side effects: blue urine; *blurred vision; dizziness; dry mouth; rapid heartbeat*

Methenamine, phenyl salicylate, methylene blue, benzoic acid, atropine sulfate, hyoscyamine
Brand: Urised (Webcon)
Tablet
Indication: urinary tract infection
Actions: reduces bacteria; relieves pain
Possible side effects: blue urine; *blurred vision; dizziness; dry mouth; rapid heartbeat*

Methenamine, sodium acid phosphate

Brand: Uro-Phosphate (Poythress)
Tablet
Indication: urinary tract infection
Action: reduces bacteria
Possible side effects: nausea; vomiting; difficult or painful urination; *rash and other allergic reactions*

Methyclothiazide. See *Cardiovascular System*

Metolazone. See *Cardiovascular System*

Metronidazole
Brand: Flagyl (Searle)
Tablet
Indication: trichomonia infections
Action: reduces trichomonia
Possible side effects: anorexia; nausea; vomiting; diarrhea; confusion; diminished coordination; insomnia; dizziness; headache; depression; dark urine; unpleasant metallic taste; *decrease in white blood cells; rash and other allergic reactions*
Warning: possible *carcinogen
Note: avoid alcohol

Miconazole nitrate
Brand: Monistat 7 (Ortho)
Cream
Indication: fungal infection of skin and vaginal tract
Action: reduces fungus
Possible side effects: cramps; headache; irritation; burning; itching; *rash and other allergic reactions*

Nalidixic acid. See *Infection*

Nitrofurantoin macrocrystals
Brand: Macrodantin (Norwich-Eaton)
Capsule
Indication: urinary tract infection
Action: reduces bacteria
Possible side effects: anorexia; nausea; vomiting; diarrhea; abdominal pain; drowsiness; dizziness; headache; brown urine; **superinfection; rash and other allergic reactions*
Note: use alcohol with extreme caution

Nystatin
Brands: Mycostatin Vaginal (Squibb), Nilstat (Lederle)
Tablet (suppository)
Indication: vaginal fungal infections
Actions: reduces fungus; treats infection
Possible side effects: irritation; burning; *rash and other allergic reactions*

Penicillin V potassium. See *Infection*

Phenazopyridine hydrochloride
Brand: Pyridium (Parke-Davis)
Tablet
Indication: pain from lower urinary tract irritations
Action: relieves pain
Possible side effects: red-orange urine; indigestion; dizziness; headache; *anemia; hepatitis; rash and other allergic reactions*

Potassium chloride. See *Cardiovascular System*

Spironolactone. See *Cardiovascular System*

Spironolactone, hydrochlorothiazide. See *Cardiovascular System*

Sulfamethoxazole. See *Infection*

Sulfanilamide, aminacrine hydrochloride, allantoin
Brand: AVC Cream (Merrell-National)
Cream, Suppository

Indication: vaginal infection
Action: reduces bacteria
Possible side effects: vaginal irritation; *rash and other allergic reactions*

Sulfathiazole, sulfacetamide, sulfabenzamide
Brand: Sultrin (Ortho)
Cream, Tablet
Indication: vaginal infection
Action: reduces bacteria
Possible side effects: vaginal irritation; *rash and other allergic reactions*

Sulfisoxazole ☐I
Brand: Gantrisin (Roche)
Tablet, Liquid, Injection
Indication: urinary tract infection
Action: reduces bacteria
Possible side effects: anorexia; nausea; vomiting; abdominal cramps; headache; depression; goiter development; *photosensitivity; *hallucinations; convulsions; *blood and *liver disorders; rash and other allergic reactions*

Sulfisoxazole, phenazopyridine hydrochloride ☐I
Brand: Azo Gantrisin (Roche)
Tablet
Indication: urinary tract infection
Actions: reduces bacteria; relieves pain when urinating
Possible side effects: anorexia; nausea; vomiting; abdominal cramps; red-orange or brown urine; dizziness; headache; depression; goiter development; *photosensitivity; *hallucinations; convulsions; anemia; hepatitis; *blood disorders; rash and other allergic reactions*
See also listings for Sulfisoxazole and Phenazopyridine hydrochloride

Tetracycline hydrochloride. See *Infection*

Triamterene, hydrochlorothiazide. See *Cardiovascular System*

Trimethoprim, sulfamethoxazole. See *Infection*

NONPRESCRIPTION DRUGS

Because Contraceptor (Schering)
Foam
Indication: decrease chance of pregnancy
Action: kills sperm

Betadine Douche (Purdue Frederick)
Liquid (for douching)
Indication: vaginal inflammation
Action: reduces bacteria and irritation

Conceptrol Birth Control Cream (Ortho)
Cream
Indication: decrease chance of pregnancy
Action: kills sperm

Conceptrol Shields (Ortho)
Latex prophylactics
Indication: decrease chance of pregnancy
Action: prevents sperm from entering vagina

Delfen Contraceptive Foam (Ortho)
Foam
Indication: decrease chance of pregnancy
Action: kills sperm

Emko, Emko Pre-Fil (Schering)
Foam
Indication: decrease chance of pregnancy

Action: kills sperm

Encare (Norwich-Eaton)

Suppository

Indication: decrease chance of pregnancy

Action: kills sperm

Herbal Diuretic Tablets (Nion)

Tablet

Indication: premenstrual fluid retention

Action: reduces premenstrual fluid retention

Koromex Contraceptive Foam (Holland-Rantos)

Foam

Indication: decreases chance of pregnancy

Action: kills sperm

Koromex[II] Contraceptive Cream, Koromex II Contraceptive Jelly (Holland-Rantos)

Cream, Gel

Indication: decrease chance of pregnancy

Action: kills sperm when used with a diaphragm

Koromex[II]-A Contraceptive Jelly (Holland-Rantos)

Gel

Indication: decrease chance of pregnancy

Action: kills sperm

Lanacane Medicated Cream (Combe)

Cream

Indication: vaginal, rectal, and skin irritation

Actions: reduces bacteria; lubricates; relieves itching and discomfort

Massengill (Beecham)

Liquid, Powder (for douching), Douche (disposable)

Indication: vaginal cleaning

Action: cleans vagina

Midol (Glenbrook)

Tablet

Indications: premenstrual tension; menstrual pain, cramps, and irritability; headache; neuralgia; low backache

Action: relieves pain and discomfort

Nylmerate[II] Solution Concentrate (Holland-Rantos)

Liquid (for douching)

Indication: vaginal cleaning

Action: cleans vagina

Odrinil Natural Diuretic (Fox)

Tablet

Indication: premenstrual fluid retention

Action: reduces premenstrual fluid retention

Ortho-Creme Contraceptive Cream, Ortho-Gynol Contraceptive Jelly (Ortho)

Cream, Gel

Indication: decrease chance of pregnancy

Action: kills sperm when used with a diaphragm

Ortho Personal Lubricant (Ortho)

Gel

Indication: lubricant for douche, rectal thermometer, tampon, enema, and intercourse

Action: lubricates

Permathene H$_2$Off (Alleghany)

Tablet

Indications: premenstrual pain; fluid retention

Actions: relieves pain; reduces fluid retention

Semicid Vaginal Contraceptive Suppositories (Whitehall)

Suppository

Indication: decrease chance of pregnancy

Action: kills sperm
Sunril Premenstrual Capsules (Schering)
Capsule
Indications: premenstrual pain; fluid retention
Actions: relieves pain; reduces fluid retention
Transi-Lube (Holland-Rantos)
Foam
Indication: lubricant for douche, rectal thermometer, tampon, enema, and intercourse
Action: lubricates
Trendar Premenstrual Tablets (Whitehall)
Tablet
Indications: premenstrual pain; fluid retention
Actions: relieves pain; reduces fluid retention
Trichotine Douche (Reed & Carnrick)
Powder, Liquid (for douching)
Indication: vaginal irritation
Action: reduces itching
Tucks Cream and Ointment (Parke-Davis)
Cream, Ointment
Indication: irritations of vaginal, nipple, and rectal area
Action: decreases irritation of genital and rectal area and nipples of nursing mothers
Tucks Premoistened Pads (Parke-Davis)
Compress
Indications: vaginal or rectal itching
Action: decreases irritation
Vagisil Feminine Itching Medication (Combe)
Cream
Indications: vaginal itching, burning, or irritation
Action: reduces bacteria

VITAMINS AND MINERALS

Vitamins are derived from living (organic) substances such as animals and plants. Minerals are derived from nonliving (inorganic) substances. Both vitamins and minerals are necessary for growth and metabolism. Since the body itself cannot produce vitamins and minerals, they should be supplied by a balanced diet. They may also be taken in tablet or capsule form if the diet is inadequate. Amounts needed differ according to age and other conditions, such as pregnancy and illness. Vitamin and mineral content in food can be diminished in storage, processing, and the cooking process.

An insufficient supply of a particular vitamin or mineral may lead to a disorder called a deficiency disease. Although it is nearly impossible to take in too much of a vitamin from the diet alone, a harmful excess of some vitamins can be ingested in pill form. Vitamin and mineral supplements, like any drugs, must be consumed with caution.

Vitamins

Vitamin A
Required for: growth, vision, skin, and mucous membranes; deficiency can cause disorders of the skin and eye, especially night blindness
Sources: animal and fish liver; cheese; milk; eggs; butter; vegetables, especially dark green and yellow; fruits, especially yellow

Vitamin B₁ (Thiamine)

Required for: carbohydrate metabolism; deficiency can cause beriberi (a nerve disorder, causing nerve inflammation, heart failure, fluid retention, nausea, vomiting, mental confusion, and brain damage)

Sources: whole grain cereals; eggs; milk; meats, especially pork and liver; green vegetables, especially peas and beans

Vitamin B₂ (Riboflavin)

Required for: metabolism of fats, carbohydrates, and proteins; deficiency can cause disorders of the mouth, lips, eye, and tongue and skin rash

Sources: meats, especially liver and kidney; poultry; fish; milk; whole grain cereals; leafy green vegetables

Niacin (B₃, Nicotinic Acid)

Required for: growth, oxygenation, vision, skin; deficiency can cause pellagra (a disorder affecting the gastrointestinal tract, skin, and nervous system), anorexia, headache, and muscular weakness

Sources: liver and kidney, poultry, fish, whole grain cereals, eggs, nuts, soybeans

Vitamin B₆ (Pyridoxine)

Required for: protein metabolism, formation of red blood cells and antibodies, functioning of central nervous system; deficiency can cause disturbances of the gastrointestinal tract, blood (including anemia), and skin

Sources: whole grain cereals; fish; eggs; meats, especially liver and kidney; bananas; nuts

Vitamin B₁₂ (Cyanocobalamin)

Required for: cell formation; deficiency can cause anemia (low blood cells, mental changes, indigestion)

Sources: liver, heart, kidney, milk, eggs, cheese, fish, oysters, clams

Pantothenic Acid

Required for: metabolism of fats and carbohydrates; deficiency can cause disorders of the skin, neuromuscular system, and gastrointestinal tract (deficiency is rare)

Sources: kidney, liver, whole grain cereals, eggs, yeast, vegetables; present in most foods

Biotin

Required for: synthesis of fatty acids, function of circulatory system, production of antibodies; deficiency can cause disorders of scalp and skin, anemia, anorexia, weakness, and muscle pains (deficiency is rare)

Sources: eggs, kidney, liver, fish, yeast, nuts, milk; present in most foods

Folic Acid (Folacin)

Required for: growth of cells; deficiency can cause anemia and weight loss

Sources: chicken, kidney, liver, yogurt, leafy green vegetables

Vitamin C (Ascorbic Acid)

Required for: a protein that forms skin, bone, and tendons; wound healing; deficiency can cause scurvy (sore gums, loosening of teeth, bleeding under skin), fatigue, diminished blood clotting, and slowed healing of wounds

Sources: fruits, especially citrus fruits; green vegetables

Vitamin D (Calciferol)

Required for: teeth and bones; deficiency can cause rickets (a bone deformity and weakness)

Sources: sun and light change cholesterol in the skin to Vitamin D; fish liver oils, enriched milk, tuna, eggs

Vitamin E (Tocopherol)
Required for: red blood cells, skeletal muscles, reproduction
Sources: whole grain cereals, meats, milk, eggs, liver, leafy green and yellow vegetables, vegetable oils

Minerals

Calcium
Required for: bones, teeth, and nerve and muscle cells; blood clotting
Sources: milk, yogurt, cheese, leafy green vegetables, molasses, soybeans, whole grain cereals

Copper
Required for: red blood cells, iron absorption
Sources: shellfish, molasses, soybeans, nuts, mushrooms, liver, kidney, heart, brain

Fluorine
Required for: making teeth resistant to decay by hardening enamel
Sources: fluoridated water (supplements insufficient amounts found in foods)

Iodine
Required for: hormones formed by thyroid gland
Sources: iodized salt, seafood, milk

Iron
Required for: transportation of oxygen to cells; deficiency can cause anemia
Sources: lean meats, especially liver, heart, kidney; shellfish; dried beans and peas; green vegetables; dried fruits; egg yolks; molasses; whole grain breads and cereals

Magnesium
Required for: metabolism, helps reduce cholesterol level
Sources: nuts, whole grain breads and cereals, eggs, milk

Phosphorus
Required for: teeth and bones, muscle contraction, nerve function
Sources: soybeans, yeast, milk, liver, eggs

Zinc
Required for: protein metabolism, skeletal growth, healing; essential constituent of several hormones
Sources: liver, nuts, oysters

Most vitamins and minerals can be acquired without a doctor's prescription and are usually left to the individual's discretion. However, some are frequently prescribed or recommended by doctors to correct or prevent the diseases that are caused by a deficiency of these vital substances. Among them are:

Vitamins A, D, C, fluoride
Brand: Tri-Vi-Flor (Mead Johnson)
Liquid, Tablet
Indications: dietary lack of vitamins; insufficient fluoride content of drinking water
Actions: supplements vitamins; prevents tooth decay
Possible side effects: rash and other allergic reactions

Vitamins A, D, E, C, B_1, B_2, B_6, B_{12}, folic acid, fluoride
Brand: Poly-Vi-Flor Chewable (Mead Johnson)

Tablet

Indications: dietary lack of vitamins; insufficient fluoride content of drinking water

Actions: supplements vitamins; prevents tooth decay

Possible side effects: rash and other allergic reactions

Ferrous sulfate

Generic manufacturers: American, Purepac

Brand: Feosol (Smith Kline & French)

Capsule, Tablet

Indications: iron deficiency; iron-deficiency anemia

Action: provides iron

Possible side effects: nausea; vomiting; constipation, diarrhea; stained teeth; dark stools

Sodium fluoride

Brands: Fluoritab (Fluoritab), Luride (Hoyt), Pediaflor (Ross)

Tablet, Liquid

Indication: insufficient fluoride content of drinking water

Actions: supplements fluoride; prevents tooth decay

Possible side effects: mottling of teeth with excess dosage

ALCOHOL, CAFFEINE, AND TOBACCO

Alcohol

For thousands of years alcohol has been used for therapeutic and psychosocial purposes. Today alcohol is used medically to stimulate appetite in the elderly and as a rubbing solution to disinfect or cool the skin. It is also used to dissolve drugs taken by mouth and is therefore an ingredient in many liquid medicines. Alcohol is used as a home remedy for "head colds," anxiety, or insomnia, but the documented therapeutic value of alcohol is limited when compared to its usage for psychosocial purposes. In the United States, two thirds of all adults use alcohol occasionally, and 15% of the users are considered "heavy drinkers."

CHEMISTRY AND METABOLISM

Ethyl alcohol is produced for commercial drinks by the fermentation of grains or fruits, as in beer or wine. The alcoholic content may then be increased if the liquid is distilled, as in whiskey or brandy. A solution with 50% alcohol is considered 100 proof. Beer contains some protein and carbohydrates, but distilled spirits contain no foodstuffs and no vitamins. Methyl alcohol, or "wood alcohol," is very dangerous because it can lead to blindness or death.

Alcohol is rapidly absorbed from the gastrointestinal tract. Food in the stomach can slow down this process. Up to 10% of the absorbed alcohol is not metabolized and is eliminated through the kidneys, lungs, and sweat glands (which is why one can "reek of alcohol"). Approximately one glass of beer, one glass of wine, or one ounce of whiskey can be metabolized by a 150-lb. adult every hour. This rate of ingestion prevents accumulation in the body, and intoxication probably will not occur. The effects of alcohol are directly related to the amount, rate of ingestion, and concentration in the blood.

ACTIONS

Nervous System. Alcohol's most noticeable effect is on the central nervous system. By depressing parts of the brain that restrain behavior, alcohol appears to have a stimulating action. In fact, mental and physical abilities are not improved, but confidence does increase and inhibitions are reduced. Higher concentrations of alcohol depress other parts of the brain until drowsiness and then sleep occur.

Cardiovascular System. Moderate doses of alcohol cause the blood vessels to dilate, producing a warm and flushed skin. Daily moderate usage (one cocktail or two beers) has been correlated with less heart disease from arteriosclerosis, but high blood pressure and heart muscle problems are associated with heavy alcohol usage.

Gastrointestinal System. Alcohol stimulates appetite and the secretions of salivary and gastric juices. Strong alcoholic drinks are irritating to the stomach's lining and cause gastritis. Chronic heavy drinking interferes with the absorption of vitamins and causes inflammation of the pancreas (pancreatitis) and of the liver (hepatitis). When the liver becomes scarred and cannot function (cirrhosis), various waste products accumulate in the body (jaundice), and fluid builds up in the abdomen and legs (ascites).

Urogenital System. Alcohol affects the fluid-regulating system in the brain as well as the kidneys so that excessive urination results. The amount excreted is greater than the amount of fluid ingested. In regard to sexual functioning, Shakespeare's statement still holds true: alcohol "provokes the desire, but it takes away the performance . . ."

CAUTIONS

Interactions with other Drugs. Because alcohol depresses the central nervous system, caution should be taken when combining alcohol with any other of the numerous drugs that have a similar depressing effect. The resulting drowsiness and mental confusion may cause overdosage, accidents, and even cessation of breathing.

Pregnancy. Alcohol directly affects the fetus. Moderate-to-heavy usage is associated with fetal malnutrition, low initial weight and length, mental retardation, hyperactivity, and birth defects. The minimum amount of alcohol to cause such problems is not known, but an intake of four or five 1-ounce drinks daily, perhaps even fewer, results in about a 12% incidence of fetal alcohol syndrome with multiple abnormalities.

Alcoholism and Alcohol Abuse. Excessive consumption of alcohol is a serious public health problem. Alcohol is involved in 30% of all suicides, 40% of all assaults, and over 50% of all fatal automobile accidents and homicides. About 10 million Americans abuse alcohol, which affects family members, employment, and medical care, and is emotionally as well as physically disastrous to the user.

The consumption of alcohol over time leads to "tolerance" so that increasing amounts of alcohol are required to produce the same "glow" or desired effect. This tolerance is associated with physical dependence, which means that withdrawal of alcohol produces tremulousness, nausea, vomiting, profuse sweating, anxiety, convulsions, and, of course, a desire to drink alcohol and relieve these distressing symptoms. These effects of physical dependency usually occur 12 to 48 hours after the last drink and may be heralded by "morning shakes." When most severe, confusion and hallucinations occur so that the individual becomes disoriented and delirious (delirium tremens, DT's) and has distorted sensations and visions (experiences bugs crawling on the skin).

Most individuals with alcoholism do not have these severe signs and go undiagnosed by family and physcians. Only 3% are skid row derelicts; most are able to hold jobs and perform basic responsibilities but their physiological, psychological, family, or social life is impaired by the use of alcohol. Because minimization, disavowal, and denial are common features of alcoholism, the disease may go unnoticed for years until physical or interpersonal problems become so severe the illness cannot be ignored. Even "blackouts" may go undetected; that is, moments or even hours may occur in the course of a day during which the individual appears to be functioning normally but later cannot recall what happened. Other types of memory loss are also caused by chronic alcohol use, which usually starts with "social" drinking.

Possible treatment approaches include detoxification, abstinence, antidepressants, group therapy, Alcoholics Anonymous, Alanon, Alateen, and employee assistance programs. Sometimes disulfiran (Antabuse) is used as well. If alcohol is consumed *in any form* (including in sauces and medication) two to five days after Antabuse is taken, an unpleasant reaction occurs with sweating, palpitations, nausea, vomiting, drowsiness, lowered blood pressure, and distressed breathing. This drug will make the impulsive drinker less likely to consume alcohol if he or she has recently taken the Antabuse. Side effects include a peculiar metallic taste, skin rash, and fatigue. A history of psychosis or heart problems are contraindications for taking Antabuse.

Caffeine

Caffeine is a stimulant obtained from different plants throughout the world. In the United States, the most common beverages containing caffeine and related stimulants are coffee, tea, cocoa, and cola-flavored drinks. Caffeine is also an ingredient in some medications including those to prevent drowsiness (for example, No Doz) and those to relieve headaches (for example, Anacin).

CHEMISTRY AND METABOLISM

Caffeine is rapidly absorbed after ingestion. One cup of coffee or tea contains about 100–150 mg of caffeine; a 12-oz. bottle of cola contains about 35–55 mg; and decaffeinated coffee contains 1–6 mg.

ACTIONS

Nervous System. Caffeine stimulates the brain to allay drowsiness and to produce clearer thinking, faster reaction time, and keen perception.

Cardiovascular System. Individuals vary in their responses to caffeine. Most have a slightly increased blood pressure and heart rate, some have a rapid or irregular heartbeat with palpitations, and some even have a slower heart rate. Whether caffeine can be used therapeutically to increase circulation in the heart and strengthen the heart muscles is controversial.

Gastrointestinal System. In usual dosages caffeine increases the secretions and motor activity of the digestive system, predisposing some individuals to gastritis, ulcers, or diarrhea.

CAUTIONS

Insomnia and Excitement. Some persons, particularly children or the elderly, are highly sensitive to the stimulating effect of caffeine and, after one cup of coffee, cannot sleep and become irritable or nervous. These individuals should be aware of drugs containing caffeine, such as medication for headaches or colds.

Abuse. Some people develop a tolerance to caffeine and overindulge to obtain the stimulating effect without being aware that their palpitations, nervousness, indigestion, heartburn, and constipation are caused by the heavy consumption of caffeine. These habituated individuals may also not realize that their morning headaches may be caused by withdrawal from caffeine and that their response to certain pain mixtures may actually be due to replenishing the caffeine. Recent evidence has indicated that heavy use of caffeine may adversely affect the development of a fetus. A pregnant woman who is inclined to overindulge in caffeine should discuss this with her doctor.

Tobacco (Nicotine)

Tobacco is the dried leaf of a plant (*Nicotiana tabacum*) that was indigenous to North America but is now grown throughout the world. About 800 billion cigarettes are smoked every year in the United States in addition to the tobacco consumed in cigars, pipes, snuffing, and chewing. No therapeutic use of tobacco or nicotine is known at this time.

CHEMISTRY AND METABOLISM

The percentage of nicotine in tobacco varies sixteenfold, from 0.5% to 8%. This variance in the leaf and the effects of different kinds of filters influence the amount of nicotine per cigarette or cigar that is absorbed; for example, the lower nicotine cigarettes may yield only 1 mg nicotine whereas some cigars may yield more than 40 mg. About 90% of nicotine is absorbed when the smoke is inhaled compared with 25%–50% when the smoke is drawn into the mouth and expelled. Therefore, more nicotine may be absorbed from an uninhaled cigar than from an inhaled low-nicotine cigarette. In addition to nicotine, tobacco smoke contains over 500 chemical compounds, including acids, irritating tars, and carbon monoxide. The pleasurable or harmful effects of tobacco use may be derived from these substances and not only from nicotine.

ACTIONS

Nervous System. Nicotine stimulates the nervous system and may cause irritability, nervousness, and tremors. An overdosage (acute nicotine poisioning) can cause confusion, cold sweats, convulsions, and paralysis of the respiratory muscles leading to death.

Cardiovascular System. Nicotine raises the blood pressure and constricts blood vessels, both of which increase the work of the heart.

Gastrointestinal System. Nicotine increases the motor activity of the intestines, causing diarrhea in susceptible individuals. Increased salivation is mainly a reaction to the smoke and not to nicotine.

CAUTIONS

Smoking is the nation's greatest public health hazard. In the United States about 400,000 people die every year because of tobacco use. Statistically, every cigarette shortens an individual's life by 14 minutes. There may also be danger to nonsmokers who breathe cigarette smoke.

Cancer. Cigarette smokers have an eleven times greater chance of having lung cancer, the most common cancer among American men. Studies have also confirmed a similar relationship between smoking and cancers of the oral cavity (mouth, lip, larynx, and esophagus).

Respiratory Diseases. Chronic tobacco smoking can lead to wheezing, shortness of breath, chest pain, and more frequent "colds" and respiratory infections. These symptoms may mimic asthma. The incidence of obstructive lung disease and emphysema is also increased. Observable damage to the lung along with respiratory symptoms can occur after only one year of a smoking habit.

Cardiovascular Diseases. Smoking tobacco significantly increases the risk of heart disease, high blood pressure, and strokes (cerebrovascular accidents).

Peptic Ulcers. The incidence of ulcers and resulting death are significantly higher in smokers.

Pregnancy. High blood pressure during pregnancy (preeclampsia), miscarriages, impaired fertility, mortality in the newly born, and lower birth weights have all been associated with cigarette smoking.

DRUG ABUSE

Any drug can be abused. This abuse may be occasional or chronic. Some drugs are more habit-forming than others because they produce a desired effect, are readily available, and are more socially acceptable. For example, the most commonly abused drugs in the United States are alcohol, caffeine, and nicotine (see preceding chapter).

Psychological dependence on a drug occurs when a person believes the drug is necessary to maintain a state of well-being and craves the drug when it is withheld. *Physical dependence* on a drug means that if the drug is stopped abruptly, a physiological withdrawal syndrome will occur, possibly causing diarrhea, anxiety attacks, tremors, or even convulsions and death. *Addiction* to a drug refers to a complex pattern of compulsive drug use characterized by an overwhelming preoccupation with taking the drug and securing its supply, combined with a strong tendency to return to this pattern after a period of being withdrawn or abstaining. A person can be addicted to a drug and not be physically dependent or be physically dependent on a drug and not be addicted (see chapter on Pain).

Most abused drugs act on the central nervous system as stimulants (cocaine, amphetamines), as depressants (alcohol, barbiturates, tranquilizers), as hallucinogens (LSD, marijuana, "angel dust"), or as narcotics (heroin, opium).

CENTRAL NERVOUS SYSTEM STIMULANTS

Amphetamines (such as Dexedrine) are taken by mouth to increase concentration and to reduce fatigue. A false sense of one's capacities may result from intoxication so that a person believes a great deal is being accomplished when in fact progress is minimal. If injected intravenously for a rapid "high," these stimulants can raise the blood pressure and cause convulsions or death.

Cocaine is either sniffed or injected intravenously (digestive juices make the drug ineffective if taken by mouth). The stimulating effect may cause heightened awareness of taste, smell, touch, sound, and vision. These effects may be fascinating or may become alarming, causing increased suspiciousness of others or a belief that bugs are crawling beneath the skin. Some users become overtly psychotic. Chronic "sniffing" can cause inflammation of the mucous membrane lining the nose.

When stimulants are discontinued, a person may experience terrifying nightmares for weeks or become profoundly depressed ("crash") to the point of feeling suicidal. This depression can increase the desire to resume taking the drug.

CENTRAL NERVOUS SYSTEM DEPRESSANTS

The nonmedical use of *barbiturates and related drugs* far exceeds the use of narcotics such as heroin. The physical risks are far more dangerous in that abrupt withdrawal after chronic use can lead to seizures, delirium, and death. If physical dependency has developed, medically supervised detoxification is advised.

The length of time required to develop physical dependence varies considerably according to the dosage, the kind of medication taken, and the individual's susceptibility. A person may be given a prescription for a drug to relieve insomnia or anxiety, then gradually increase the dosage at night, and begin taking a pill or two in the morning to "relax" until the drug is a major part of the user's life and higher and higher dosages are required to produce the desired calming effect. Personality changes, hostility, irritability, irresponsibility, untidiness, slurred speech, and depression may accompany this decline.

CENTRAL NERVOUS SYSTEM HALLUCINOGENS

Hallucinogens (psychedelics) produce perceptual distortions and profound changes in mood without marked changes in consciousness. Other kinds of drugs affecting the nervous system can also cause such distortions, but psychedelics uniformly induce a state otherwise only experienced in dreams.

The effect of an hallucinogen will depend on the individual's susceptibility, previous drug usage, expectations, and surroundings as well as the kind and amount of hallucinogen taken. With *LSD*, for example, the user may experience, within a few minutes, dizziness followed by an inner tension that is relieved by laughing or crying until several feelings seem to coexist at the same time. During the second hour the user may have even less of a sense of control over what is being experienced and may feel like a mere observer. The body appears distorted with poorly demarcated boundaries. Colors are thought to be "tasted," and time may seem to stop. Such distortions may contribute to what the user experiences as a feeling of harmony filled with "cosmic meaning" as the mind becomes "expanded."

The distortions and fragmentation may also produce a panic reaction, psychosis, profound depression, and impulsive acts, such as suicide. These "bad trips" may last 24 hours and may occur in users who previously had experienced only "good trips." Some susceptible individuals have "flashbacks," recurrences of the drug effects days or weeks later without the drug.

Another psychedelic drug, *DMT* is not active if taken by mouth, so it is usually inhaled as a powder or sprinkled over

Drug Abuse

Type (common names)	Effects	Risks
Stimulants amphetamines (uppers, speed, crystal) Dexadrine (dexies) Benzedrine (bennies) cocaine (coke, dust)	increased energy and concentration rapid heartbeat heightened perceptions hallucinations	hyperactivity hypertension psychosis paranoia strokes *withdrawal may produce:* fatigue, depression, nightmares, suicide
Depressants alcohol barbiturates (goof balls, reds, yellow jackets, red devils) anti-anxiety drugs chlordiazepoxide—Librium chlorazepate—Tranxene diazepam—Valium meprobamate—Equanil, Miltown oxazepam—Serax hypnotics (sleeping pills) ethchlorvynol—Placidyl glutethimide—Doriden methaqualone (soaps, downers) pentobarbital—Nembutol (yellow jacket) secobarbital (red devils)—Seconal	sedation lethargy decreased attention sluggish thinking gait imbalance	irrationality impulsivity hostility paranoia personality changes psychosis *withdrawal may produce:* tremulousness, hallucinations, seizures, delusions, death
Hallucinogens (psychedelics) atropine D-lysergic acid diethylamide (LSD, acid) mescaline; peyote N.N dimethyltryptamine (DMT, business man's trip) phencyclidine (angel dust, PCP, hog, peace pill) psilocybin 2g5-dimethoxy-4-methylamphetamine (DOM, STP) scopalomine (in nonprescription sleeping pills)	perceptual distortions hallucinations altered mood, thinking, and behavior diminished control over imagination sense of spiritual exaltation	psychosis panic attacks "bad trips" "flashbacks" convulsions fetal abnormalities suicide or death
Cannabinoids marijuana (grass, pot, Acapulco Gold) hashish (hash)	sense of relaxation and well-being	decreased motivation
Narcotics codeine heroin (junk, snow, H, bag) meperidine—Demerol methadone morphine (dope)	drowsiness orgasm-like "rush" emotional detachment constricted pupils constipation decreased libido	respiratory depression infected veins, skin, blood, brain, kidneys, heart valves allergic reaction to impurities death from overdose *withdrawal may produce:* abdominal cramps, runny nose, diarrhea, "gooseflesh," chills, tremulousness

tobacco, producing a rapid "trip" lasting for only one or two hours. *PCP* (angel dust) is also inhaled, often sprinkled over marijuana. This highly dangerous drug can produce convulsions, coma, and death. Unless extremely concentrated, *marijuana* or *hashish* usually do not produce profound distortions; a heightened perceptual awareness may occur and events become invested with significant positive or negative emotional feelings. Occasionally, users will experience a panic attack and become psychotically paranoid. Chronic marijuana use has been associated with continuing lethargy, social withdrawal, and a lack of interest in work ("amotivational syndrome"). In search of different drug experiences, "basement chemists" have produced a variety of psychedelics, and the ingredients are not always known by the user.

CENTRAL NERVOUS SYSTEM NARCOTICS

Most adults in the United States have taken narcotics, such as *codeine, morphine,* and *meperidine* (Demerol) at some time or other during their lives. After the medical reason for taking these drugs has passed, almost all patients then discontinue taking the drug and have no craving for it. Similarly, people can experiment with narcotics "recreationally" and not become physically dependent or addicted. Why some individuals go on to become compulsive users is not well understood.

Narcotics relieve pain, dull sensation, and induce sleep. Although alleged to produce euphoria, when first taken, narcotics, such as heroin and morphine, more commonly produce an unpleasant "dopiness" with nausea and even vomiting. Some people, however, discover a new world of satisfaction and decide to use the drug as frequently as finances will permit. A rapid intravenous injection of a narcotic induces a warm flushing of the skin and a sensation in the lower abdomen similar to sexual orgasm. This sensation, called a "rush" or "kick," is followed by a dreamy indifference, a "high," which may last for two to six hours while the user is "on the nod." The user may then wish to repeat this experience with another injection of heroin or morphine or may be driven to take another dosage before distressing withdrawal symptoms occur in about twelve to twenty-four hours. With methadone, however, the effects tend to last longer and the withdrawal syndrome is more gradual. Withdrawal symptoms include restlessness, increased perspiring, abdominal and muscle cramps, running nose, and chills. Unlike withdrawal from alcohol, barbiturates, and some tranquilizers, withdrawal from narcotics is rarely fatal. Babies born to mothers who have been taking narcotics regularly prior to delivery will be physically dependent and have withdrawal symptoms.

Along with the psychosocial problems of continual narcotic usage, medical problems include severe constipation, impotence and loss of libido, infection of the skin, blood, kidneys, brain, and heart valves as a result of unsterile injections, and toxic or allergic reactions to substances with which the narcotic is mixed. An overdosage can stop respiration and lead to death. This overdosage may be inadvertent, occurring because the user did not know the strength or purity of the drug. An emergency injection of naloxone, a narcotic antagonist, can block the potentially fatal effects of a narcotic and can also lead to a withdrawal syndrome.

DRUG PRECAUTIONS

The top of the chart lists common situations or illnesses that require special consideration before a drug is taken. A • beside the listed prescription drug does not mean that the drug should not be taken under these conditions, but does indicate that special precaution is necessary and that consultation with a doctor or pharmacist is advisable. An alternative drug or a smaller dosage may be indicated.

	Using Alcohol or Tranquilizers	Pregnant or Nursing	Of Advanced Age	High Blood Pressure	Heart Disease	Kidney/Liver Disease	Ulcers	Glaucoma	Diabetes	Epilepsy	Sun Exposure	Operating Machinery
ACHROMYCIN	•	•	•	•				•			•	
ACTIFED	•	•	•	•	•	•	•		•	•	•	•
ACTIFED-C EXPECTORANT	•	•	•	•	•	•	•	•	•	•		•
ADAPIN	•	•	•	•				•	•	•	•	•
ADRIAMYCIN	•	•				•	•					
ADROYD	•			•		•	•		•			
ADRUCIL INJECTABLE	•	•				•						
AEROLONE	•			•		•	•					
ALDACTAZIDE	•	•	•	•		•			•		•	•
ALDACTONE	•	•		•		•						
ALDOMET	•	•	•	•		•			•			•
ALDORIL	•	•	•	•		•			•		•	•
ALKERAN	•	•										
ALUPENT	•			•		•	•		•			
AMBENYL EXPECTORANT	•	•	•	•	•	•	•		•		•	•
AMCILL	•	•		•								
AMINOPHYLLIN	•	•		•	•	•	•	•				
AMOXICILLIN	•	•		•								
AMOXIL	•	•		•								
AMPHICOL	•	•	•	•				•				
AMPICILLIN	•	•		•								
ANADROL-50	•			•		•	•		•			
ANTEPAR	•	•				•				•		
ANTIBIOPTO	•	•	•	•		•						
ANTIMINTH	•	•				•						
ANTIVERT	•	•	•	•								•
ANUSOL-HC	•			•				•				
APOMORPHINE HYDROCHLORIDE	•	•	•	•			•					
APRESOLINE HYDROCHLORIDE	•	•	•	•		•	•					•
ARALEN	•	•				•						
ARISTOCORT	•	•		•	•	•			•	•		

	USING ALCOHOL OR TRANQUILIZERS	PREGNANT	NURSING	OF ADVANCED AGE	HIGH BLOOD PRESSURE	ULCERS	KIDNEY/LIVER DISEASE	HEART DISEASE	GLAUCOMA	DIABETES	EPILEPSY	OPERATING MACHINERY	SUN EXPOSURE
ARMOUR THYROID				•			•	•			•		
ARTANE	•	•	•	•		•	•	•	•				•
ATARAX	•	•	•	•					•		•		•
ATIVAN	•	•	•	•			•	•					•
ATROMID-S	•	•		•	•		•		•				•
AVC CREAM	•												
AVENTYL	•	•	•	•			•		•	•	•	•	•
AZO GANTRISIN	•	•	•	•			•		•		•		
AZULFIDINE	•	•	•	•			•		•		•		
BACTRIM	•	•	•	•			•		•		•		
BACTRIM DS	•	•	•	•			•		•		•		
BENADRYL	•	•	•	•	•	•	•		•			•	•
BENDECTIN	•	•	•	•	•				•				•
BENEMID	•	•		•	•			•					
BENTYL	•	•		•	•		•	•	•				•
BENYLIN COUGH SYRUP	•	•	•	•	•	•	•		•		•	•	•
BICNU	•	•											
BRETHINE	•	•		•		•	•			•	•		
BUTAZOLIDIN	•	•		•	•		•	•		•	•		•
BUTAZOLIDIN ALKA	•	•		•	•		•	•		•	•		•
BUTICAPS	•	•	•	•			•			•	•	•	
BUTISOL SODIUM	•	•	•	•			•			•	•	•	
CANDEX													
CARBARSONE									•				
CATAPRES	•	•	•	•			•	•					•
CEENU	•	•											
CELESTONE	•	•				•	•		•	•			
CHLOROMYCETIN	•	•	•	•			•						
CHLOROMYCETIN OPHTHALMIC													
CHLOROMYCETIN OTIC													
CHLOROPTIC	•	•	•	•			•						
CHLOR-TRIMETON REPETABS	•	•	•	•	•	•	•		•				•
CHOLEDYL	•	•		•	•	•	•	•					
CLEOCIN HYDROCHLORIDE	•	•		•			•						
CLINORIL	•	•			•	•	•	•					
COGENTIN	•	•		•		•	•	•	•				•
COLCHICINE	•	•		•			•	•					
COLY-MYCIN S OTIC													
COMBID	•	•	•	•	•		•	•	•		•	•	•
COMPAZINE	•	•	•	•	•	•	•	•	•		•	•	•
CORDRAN	•												
CORTEF	•	•		•	•	•		•	•	•			

	USING ALCOHOL OR TRANQUILIZERS	OF ADVANCED AGE	NURSING	PREGNANT	HIGH BLOOD PRESSURE	KIDNEY/LIVER DISEASE	HEART DISEASE	ULCERS	GLAUCOMA	DIABETES	SUN EXPOSURE	EPILEPSY	OPERATING MACHINERY
CORTENEMA	•	•		•	•	•		•	•	•			
CORTISPORIN OPHTHALMIC													
CORTISPORIN OTIC													
CORTRIL	•	•		•	•	•		•	•	•			
COSMEGEN	•	•								•			
COUMADIN	•	•	•	•	•	•	•	•		•		•	
CUPRIMINE	•	•		•						•			
CYCLOSPASMOL	•	•		•			•			•			
CYTOMEL				•		•	•			•			
DALMANE	•	•	•	•		•					•		•
DANOCRINE	•	•		•			•	•			•		
DAPSONE	•	•		•									
DARAPRIM	•	•									•		
DARVOCET-N 50	•	•	•	•	•								•
DARVOCET-N 100	•	•	•	•	•								•
DARVON	•	•	•	•	•								•
DARVON COMPOUND-65	•	•	•	•	•								•
DECADRON	•	•	•	•	•	•			•	•			
DELTASONE	•	•		•	•	•			•	•			
DEMEROL	•	•	•	•			•	•			•		•
DEMULEN	•	•				•	•	•		•	•	•	
DEPEN TITRATABS	•	•		•				•					
DEPO-PROVERA	•	•				•	•	•		•	•		
DEXAMETHASONE	•	•	•	•	•	•			•	•			
DEXEDRINE	•	•	•	•		•	•	•		•	•		•
DIABINESE	•	•	•	•	•			•		•		•	•
DIAMOX	•	•		•			•	•					
DIETHYLSTILBESTROL	•	•		•		•	•	•		•	•	•	
DIGITOXIN	•	•		•			•	•					
DIGOXIN	•	•		•			•	•					
DILANTIN	•	•	•	•			•	•		•	•	•	•
DIMETANE EXPECTORANT	•	•	•	•	•	•	•		•	•			•
DIMETANE EXPECTORANT-DC	•	•	•	•	•	•	•	•	•	•			•
DIMETANE EXTENTABS	•	•	•	•	•	•	•		•				•
DIMETAPP	•	•	•	•	•	•	•		•	•			•
DIUPRES	•	•	•	•			•			•		•	•
DIURIL	•	•	•	•			•			•		•	•
DOLOPHINE HYDROCHLORIDE	•	•	•	•			•						•
DONNATAL	•	•	•	•	•		•	•	•	•		•	•
DORIDEN	•	•	•	•									•
DRIXORAL	•	•	•	•		•	•		•	•			•
DROLBAN	•	•					•						
DTIC-DOME	•	•							•				

	PREGNANT	NURSING	USING ALCOHOL OR TRANQUILIZERS	OF ADVANCED AGE	HIGH BLOOD PRESSURE	KIDNEY/LIVER DISEASE	HEART DISEASE	ULCERS	GLAUCOMA	DIABETES	EPILEPSY	SUN EXPOSURE	OPERATING MACHINERY
DYAZIDE	•	•	•	•				•		•		•	•
DYMELOR	•	•	•	•	•			•		•		•	•
DYNAPEN	•	•					•	•					
ECONOCHLOR	•	•	•	•				•					
E.E.S.	•	•	•	•				•					
EFUDEX	•												
ELAVIL	•	•	•	•			•		•	•	•	•	•
ELIXOPHYLLIN	•	•			•	•	•	•	•				
ELSPAR	•	•						•					
EMPIRIN WITH CODEINE	•	•	•	•	•			•					•
EMPRACET	•	•	•	•	•			•					•
E-MYCIN	•	•	•	•				•					
ENDURON	•	•	•	•				•				•	•
EPINEPHRINE HYDROCHLORIDE	•		•	•		•	•		•	•			
EQUAGESIC	•	•	•	•	•			•		•	•		•
EQUANIL	•	•	•	•				•			•		•
ERYTHROCIN	•	•	•	•				•					
ERYTHROMYCIN	•	•	•	•				•					
ESIDRIX	•	•	•	•				•		•		•	•
ESKALITH	•	•	•	•			•	•		•	•		•
ESTINYL	•	•				•	•	•		•	•		
FASTIN	•	•	•	•			•	•		•	•		•
FEOSOL													
FERROUS SULFATE													
FIORINAL	•	•	•	•	•		•	•		•	•	•	•
FIORINAL WITH CODEINE	•	•	•	•	•		•	•		•	•	•	•
FLAGYL	•	•	•	•									•
FLEXERIL	•	•	•				•		•				•
FLORINEF ACETATE	•	•		•	•	•	•	•		•	•		
FLURORITAB													
FUDR	•	•						•					
FULVICIN	•	•	•	•				•			•		
FUNGIZONE													
GANTANOL	•	•	•	•				•		•		•	
GANTRISIN	•	•	•	•				•		•		•	
GANTRISIN OPHTHALMIC													
GARAMYCIN													
GARAMYCIN OPHTHALMIC													
GEOCILLIN	•	•						•					
GRIFULVIN V	•	•	•	•				•			•		
GRISACTIN	•	•	•	•				•			•		
GRIS-PEG	•	•	•	•				•			•		
GYNE-LOTRIMIN	•												
HALDOL	•	•	•	•		•	•	•	•	•	•	•	•

	Using Alcohol or Tranquilizers	Pregnant	Nursing	Of Advanced Age	High Blood Pressure	Ulcers	Kidney/Liver Disease	Heart Disease	Glaucoma	Diabetes	Epilepsy	Operating Machinery	Sun Exposure
HYDERGINE			•	•		•							
HYDROCHLOROTHIAZIDE	•	•		•				•		•		•	•
HYDROCORTONE	•	•		•	•	•		•	•	•			
HYDRODIURIL	•	•	•	•				•		•		•	•
HYDROPRES	•	•	•	•	•			•		•	•	•	•
HYGROTON	•	•	•	•				•		•		•	•
ILETIN LENTE	•		•	•									
ILOSONE	•	•	•	•			•						
INDERAL	•	•	•	•			•	•		•			•
INDOCIN	•	•		•	•	•					•		•
INH	•	•	•					•		•	•		
INSULIN NPH	•		•	•									
IONAMIN	•	•	•	•		•	•		•	•			•
IPECAC	•	•											
ISMELIN	•	•	•	•	•		•			•			•
ISOPHANE INSULIN	•		•	•									
ISOPTO-CARPINE	•	•	•										
ISORDIL	•	•	•	•					•				
KANTREX	•	•						•					
KEFLEX	•	•		•				•					
KENALOG	•												
KENALOG IN ORABASE	•					•				•			
K-LYTE		•		•	•	•	•	•		•			
KWELL	•												
LANOXIN	•	•		•			•	•					
LAROTID	•	•		•									
LASIX ORAL	•	•	•	•				•		•			•
LEUKERAN	•	•											
LEVODOPA	•	•		•	•	•	•	•	•	•	•		•
LEVO-DROMORAN	•	•	•	•									
LEVOTHROID				•	•		•	•		•			
LIBRAX	•	•	•	•			•	•	•	•	•	•	•
LIBRIUM	•	•	•	•						•	•	•	•
LIDEX	•												
LINCOCIN	•	•		•				•					
LIORESAL	•	•	•	•				•			•		•
LITHANE	•	•	•	•			•	•		•	•		•
LITHIUM CARBONATE	•	•	•	•			•	•		•	•		•
LITHOBID	•	•	•	•			•	•		•	•		•
LITHONATE	•	•	•	•			•	•		•	•		•
LITHOTABS	•	•	•	•			•	•		•	•		•
LOMOTIL	•	•	•	•	•		•	•	•				•
LO/OVRAL	•	•				•	•	•		•	•	•	
LOPRESSOR	•	•		•	•		•	•		•		•	

	USING ALCOHOL OR TRANQUILIZERS	PREGNANT	NURSING	OF ADVANCED AGE	HIGH BLOOD PRESSURE	HEART DISEASE	KIDNEY/LIVER DISEASE	ULCERS	GLAUCOMA	DIABETES	EPILEPSY	SUN EXPOSURE	OPERATING MACHINERY
LOTRIMIN	•												
LURIDE													
LYSODREN	•	•							•				•
MACRODANTIN	•	•	•	•					•		•		
MARAX	•	•	•	•	•	•	•	•	•		•		•
MEDROL (ORAL)	•	•		•	•	•			•	•			
MELLARIL	•	•	•	•		•	•				•	•	•
MEPROBAMATE	•	•	•	•					•		•		•
METANDREN	•	•		•		•	•	•	•		•		
METHOTREXATE	•	•	•	•	•				•				
METICORTEN	•	•		•	•	•				•	•		
METIMYD													
METRETON	•												
MILTOWN	•	•	•	•					•		•		•
MILTOWN 600	•	•	•	•					•		•		•
MINIPRESS	•	•	•	•			•	•	•				
MINOCIN	•	•	•	•					•			•	•
MITHRACIN									•				
MONISTAT 7	•												
MOTRIN	•	•				•		•					
MUSTARGEN	•	•							•				
MUTAMYCIN	•	•							•				
MYAMBUTOL	•	•		•					•				
MYCHEL	•	•	•	•					•				
MYCOLOG	•												
MYCOSTATIN VAGINAL													
MYSOLINE	•	•	•	•					•				•
NAFCIL	•	•						•	•				
NALDECON	•	•		•		•	•		•	•			•
NALFON	•	•	•		•	•		•					•
NAPROSYN	•	•			•			•	•				
NAVANE	•	•	•	•		•	•	•	•	•		•	•
NEG GRAM	•	•	•						•		•	•	
NEMBUTAL ELIXIR	•	•	•	•					•		•	•	•
NEOPOLYCIN OPHTHALMIC													
NEOSPORIN OPHTHALMIC													
NICALEX	•	•	•	•	•				•		•		
NICOBID	•	•	•	•	•				•		•		
NICOLAR	•	•	•	•	•				•		•		
NICO-SPAN	•	•	•	•	•				•		•		
NICOTINEX	•	•	•	•	•				•		•		
NILSTAT LIQUID													
NILSTAT LIQUID/OINTMENT/CREAM													

	Using Alcohol or Tranquilizers	Pregnant	Nursing	Of Advanced Age	High Blood Pressure	Heart Disease	Kidney/Liver Disease	Ulcers	Glaucoma	Diabetes	Epilepsy	Operating Machinery	Sun Exposure
NILSTAT VAGINAL TABLETS													
NITRO-BID	•	•	•	•			•		•				
NITROGLYCERIN	•	•	•	•			•		•				
NITROSTAT	•	•	•	•			•		•				
NOLVADEX	•	•											
NORFLEX	•	•	•	•	•		•		•			•	
NORGESIC	•	•	•	•	•		•		•			•	
NORGESIC FORTE	•	•	•	•	•		•		•			•	
NORINYL 1 + 50 21-DAY	•	•					•	•	•		•	•	•
NORLESTRIN 1/50-21	•	•					•	•	•		•	•	•
NORLUTATE	•	•					•	•	•		•	•	•
NORPACE	•	•		•					•	•	•		
NPH ILETIN	•		•	•									
NYDRAZID	•	•	•				•			•	•		
OMNIPEN	•	•		•									
ONCOVIN	•	•							•				
OPHTHOCHLOR	•	•	•	•					•				
OPTIMYD													
ORABASE HCA	•					•						•	
ORETON METHYL	•	•		•		•	•	•			•		
ORINASE	•	•	•	•	•				•		•	•	•
ORNADE	•	•	•	•	•	•	•		•	•			•
ORTHO-NOVUM 1/80-21	•	•					•	•	•		•	•	•
ORTHO-NOVUM 1/50-28	•	•					•	•	•		•	•	•
ORTHO-NOVUM 1/50-21	•	•					•	•	•		•	•	•
OTIC-NEO-CORT-DOME													
OVRAL	•	•					•	•	•		•	•	•
OVRAL-28	•	•					•	•	•		•	•	•
OVULEN-21	•	•					•	•	•		•	•	•
OXALID	•	•	•	•	•	•	•	•	•	•		•	•
PARACORT	•	•			•	•	•			•	•		
PARAFLEX	•	•	•	•			•					•	
PARAFON FORTE	•	•	•	•			•					•	
PAREDRINE 1%	•								•		•	•	
PAREGORIC	•	•	•	•			•						
PAREPECTOLIN	•	•	•	•			•						
PARNATE	•	•	•	•		•	•	•		•	•	•	•
PATHOCIL	•	•					•	•					
PAVABID	•	•	•	•				•	•			•	
PBZ	•	•	•	•	•	•	•		•			•	
PEDIAFLOR													
PEDIAMYCIN	•	•	•	•			•						
PENICILLIN G POTASSIUM		•		•			•	•					
PENICILLIN VK		•		•			•	•					

	USING ALCOHOL OR TRANQUILIZERS	PREGNANT	NURSING	OF ADVANCED AGE	HIGH BLOOD PRESSURE	HEART DISEASE	KIDNEY/LIVER DISEASE	ULCERS	GLAUCOMA	DIABETES	EPILEPSY	SUN EXPOSURE	OPERATING MACHINERY
PENTIDS		•		•					•	•			
PEN-VEE K		•		•					•	•			
PERCOCET-5	•	•	•	•					•				•
PERCODAN	•	•	•	•	•								•
PERIACTIN	•	•	•	•	•	•	•			•			•
PERSANTINE	•	•	•	•				•	•				
PHAZYME-PB	•	•	•	•					•			•	•	•
PHENAPHEN WITH CODEINE	•	•	•	•					•				•
PHENERGAN EXPECTORANT	•	•	•	•	•	•		•		•			•	•
PHENERGAN EXPECTORANT WITH CODEINE	•	•	•	•	•	•	•	•	•	•			•	•
PHENERGAN VC EXPECTORANT	•	•	•	•	•	•	•	•	•	•			•	•
PHENERGAN VC EXPECTORANT WITH CODEINE	•	•	•	•	•	•	•	•	•	•			•	•
PHENOBARBITAL	•	•	•	•					•			•	•	•
PHOSPHOLINE IODINE	•					•		•		•		•	
PLACIDYL	•	•	•	•					•				•
PLATINOL	•	•							•				
POLARAMINE TABS	•	•	•	•						•			•
POLYCILLIN	•	•		•									
POLYMOX	•	•		•									
POLYSPORIN OINTMENT OPHTHALMIC													
POLY-VI-FLOR CHEWABLE													
POTASSIUM CHLORIDE		•		•	•	•	•	•	•		•		
PREDNISONE ORAL	•	•		•	•	•			•	•			
PREMARIN ORAL	•	•		•		•	•	•		•	•	•	
PRINCIPEN	•	•		•									
PRO-BANTHINE	•	•		•	•		•	•	•				•
PROCAINAMIDE HYDROCHLORIDE	•	•		•			•	•					
PROGLYCEM	•	•		•			•			•			
PROLOID				•		•	•	•		•			
PRONESTYL	•	•		•			•	•					
PROPYLTHIOURACIL	•	•		•									
PROTAMINE, ZINC & ILETIN	•		•	•									
PROVERA	•	•				•	•	•			•	•	
PURINETHOL	•	•						•					
PYRIDIUM	•	•		•									
QUESTRAN	•	•		•									
QUIBRON	•	•		•	•	•	•	•					

	USING ALCOHOL OR TRANQUILIZERS	OF ADVANCED AGE	NURSING	PREGNANT	HIGH BLOOD PRESSURE	KIDNEY/LIVER DISEASE	HEART DISEASE	ULCERS	GLAUCOMA	DIABETES	EPILEPSY	OPERATING MACHINERY	SUN EXPOSURE
QUINAMM	•		•	•									
QUINIDINE SULFATE	•	•		•			•						
REGITINE	•	•		•									
REGROTON	•	•	•	•	•					•	•	•	•
RESERPINE	•	•	•	•	•						•		•
RIFADIN	•	•	•	•					•				
RIMACTANE	•	•	•	•					•				
RITALIN	•	•	•	•					•		•		
ROBAXIN	•	•	•	•					•		•		•
ROBAXIN-750	•	•	•	•					•		•		•
SALUTENSIN	•	•	•	•	•				•		•	•	•
SANSERT	•	•		•	•	•	•		•				
SECONAL	•	•	•	•					•		•	•	•
SEPTRA	•	•	•	•					•		•		•
SEPTRA DS	•	•	•	•					•		•		•
SER-AP-ES	•	•	•	•	•				•		•	•	•
SERAX	•	•	•	•							•		•
SEROMYCIN	•	•	•						•		•		
SILVER NITRATE													
SINEQUAN	•	•	•	•			•		•		•	•	•
SK-DIGOXIN	•	•		•			•	•	•				
SKELAXIN	•	•		•					•				
SK-NIACIN	•	•	•	•	•				•		•		
SLOW-K		•		•	•	•	•	•	•		•		
SOMA	•	•		•									•
SORBITRATE	•	•	•	•						•			
S-P-T					•		•	•			•		
STELAZINE	•	•	•	•					•	•	•		•
STILPHOSTROL							•	•			•	•	
STOXIL	•	•											
SULTRIN	•								•				
SUMYCIN	•	•	•	•					•			•	
SYMMETREL	•	•	•	•	•				•	•		•	•
SYNALAR	•												
SYNALGOS-DC	•	•	•	•	•				•	•			•
SYNTHROID				•		•	•				•		
TACE	•	•					•	•	•	•		•	•
TAGAMET	•	•		•					•				•
TALWIN 50	•	•	•	•					•	•		•	•
TANDEARIL	•	•	•	•	•	•	•	•	•	•		•	•
TAPAZOLE	•	•		•									
TEDRAL	•	•	•	•	•	•	•	•	•				
TEDRAL EXPECTORANT	•	•	•	•	•	•	•	•	•				
TEDRAL SA	•	•	•	•	•	•	•	•	•				

	USING ALCOHOL OR TRANQUILIZERS	PREGNANT	NURSING	OF ADVANCED AGE	HIGH BLOOD PRESSURE	HEART DISEASE	KIDNEY/LIVER DISEASE	ULCERS	GLAUCOMA	DIABETES	EPILEPSY	SUN EXPOSURE	OPERATING MACHINERY
TEDRAL-25	•	•	•	•	•	•	•	•	•				
TEGRETOL	•	•	•	•		•	•	•	•			•	•
TENUATE	•	•	•	•		•	•		•		•		•
TESLAC	•	•											
TETRACYCLINE HYDROCHLORIDE	•	•	•	•				•				•	
TETRACYN	•	•	•	•				•				•	
THORAZINE	•	•	•	•	•		•	•	•		•	•	•
THYROID STRONG				•		•	•			•			
TIGAN	•	•	•	•				•					•
TIMOPTIC	•	•						•		•			
TOFRANIL	•	•	•	•				•		•	•	•	•
TOLECTIN	•	•	•	•	•		•	•					•
TOLECTIN DS	•	•	•	•	•		•	•					•
TOLINASE	•	•	•	•	•			•		•		•	•
TOPSYN	•												
TRAC TABS	•	•		•	•		•	•	•				•
TRANXENE	•	•	•	•					•		•		
TRIAVIL	•	•	•	•			•	•	•	•	•	•	•
TRILAFON	•	•	•	•				•			•	•	•
TRI-VI-FLOR													
TUSS-ORNADE	•	•	•	•	•	•	•	•	•	•			
TYLENOL WITH CODEINE	•	•	•	•				•					•
UNIPEN	•	•					•	•					
URISED	•	•	•	•	•		•	•	•				•
URO-PHOSPHATE	•												
VALISONE	•												
VALIUM	•	•	•	•						•	•	•	•
VANCERIL	•	•		•									
VANCOCIN				•					•				
VASODILAN	•	•		•		•							•
V-CILLIN K		•		•			•	•					
VELBAN	•	•											
VERACILLIN	•	•					•	•					
VERMOX	•	•											
VIBRAMYCIN	•	•	•	•				•				•	
VIOFORM-HYDROCORTISONE	•												
VIRA-A	•	•											
VISTARIL	•	•	•	•							•		•
VYTONE CREAM	•												
WYMOX	•	•		•									
ZAROXOLYN	•	•	•	•				•		•			
ZOMAX	•	•		•	•	•	•	•					•
ZYLOPRIM	•	•		•				•					•

CONTENTS OF
HOME MEDICINE CABINET

Indication	Action	Medication
fever; pain	analgesic;antipyretic	aspirin; acetaminophen
acid indigestion	antacid	aluminum-magnesium
diarrhea	antidiarrheal	kaolin-pectin
itching	antipruritic	calamine lotion; hydrocortisone ointment .5%
cut or abrasion	antiseptic	tincture of iodine; hydrogen peroxide
cold; flu; allergy	decongestant (nasal)	nose drops/spray with phenylephrine hydrochloride; oral with phenylpropanolamine hydrochloride
constipation	laxative	glycerine suppositories; magnesium citrate; methylcellulose
cold; flu	cough	mixture or lozenge with dextromethorphan
prevention of infection	antibiotic	neomycin-bacitracin-polymyxin B
sun exposure	sunscreen	cream or lotion with PABA
cold; flu; allergy; insect bite	antihistamine	chlorpheniramine
accidental poisoning	antidote to be taken on doctor's recommendation	ipecac; activated charcoal

EQUIPMENT

scissors	heating pad	gauze pads
oral thermometer	ice bag	cotton balls
rectal thermometer	measuring spoon	adhesive tape
hot water bottle	adhesive bandages	elastic bandage
tweezers	petroleum jelly	tongue depressors

EMERGENCY TELEPHONE NUMBERS

Town Emergency No.: _____

Poison Control: _____ Ambulance: _____

Doctor: _____

PATIENT'S PRESCRIPTION AND IMMUNIZATION RECORD

Prescriptions

Drug	Pharmacy & Prescription Number	Date Taken	Prescribed By	Prescribed For	Reaction or Allergy
1					
2					
3					
4					
5					
6					

Immunizations

Vaccine	Given To (Patient)	Given By (Doctor)	Date Taken	Next Due	Reaction
1					
2					
3					
4					
5					
6					

FAMILY MEDICAL HISTORY

It is important to keep a careful record of your family's medical history. This chart is designed to provide information that will be vital to your doctor and helpful to you, for example, when applying for health insurance. Be sure to include the common hereditary diseases, such as diabetes, heart disease, high blood pressure, bleeding disorders, and stroke, as well as dates of illnesses, surgery, and x-rays.

Name						
Date of Birth						
Blood Type						
Illness	Type	Date	Type	Date	Type	Date
Allergies	Type	Date	Type	Date	Type	Date
Surgery	Type	Date	Type	Date	Type	Date
X-Rays	Type	Date	Type	Date	Type	Date

Name						
Date of Birth						
Blood Type						
Illness	Type	Date	Type	Date	Type	Date
Allergies	Type	Date	Type	Date	Type	Date
Surgery	Type	Date	Type	Date	Type	Date
X-Rays	Type	Date	Type	Date	Type	Date

Medical Insurance:
Company & Policy No.: _____

Company & Policy No.: _____

Company & Policy No.: _____

INDEX